Psychoanalysis and Catholicism

In *Psychoanalysis and Catholicism: From Freud to Francis*, Adam J. Schneider explores the censored history of psychoanalysis by the Catholic Church, reopening dialogue on key overlapping concepts to address contemporary needs.

This book is organized into three parts. First, Schneider explores the historical relationship between psychoanalysis and the Church through key figures such as Sigmund Freud and Pope Pius XII. He then brings into conversation significant theological doctrines and psychoanalytic concepts including censorship/repression, original sin/unconscious desire, and the power of speech as examples of the fruitfulness of this dialogue. Finally, he applies theory and theology to contemporary issues like priestly and psychoanalytic formation and synodality within Lacan's four discourses. Schneider centers Pope Francis, whose papacy was a pastoral practice which reflected psychoanalytic ethics, as an orienting influence throughout the text.

Psychoanalysis and Catholicism will be of interest to readers seeking to understand how psychoanalysis and Catholicism edify one another, and how to apply these insights to clinical settings, seminary formation, and parish life.

Adam J. Schneider, PhD, is a psychologist and supervisor in Washington State, USA. He works for the Department of Corrections and is Adjunct Faculty at The Seattle School of Theology & Psychology. He has published in *Integratus, Psychoanalytische Perspectieven, Psychosis*, and the *Journal of Medical Humanities.*

Psychoanalysis and Catholicism

From Freud to Francis

Adam J. Schneider

Routledge
Taylor & Francis Group
LONDON AND NEW YORK

Designed cover image: Michal Ludwiczak / Getty Images®

First published 2026
by Routledge
4 Park Square, Milton Park, Abingdon, Oxon OX14 4RN

and by Routledge
605 Third Avenue, New York, NY 10158

Routledge is an imprint of the Taylor & Francis Group, an informa business

British Library Cataloguing-in-Publication Data
A catalogue record for this book is available from the British Library

ISBN: 978-1-032-77907-2 (hbk)
ISBN: 978-1-032-77906-5 (pbk)
ISBN: 978-1-003-48534-6 (ebk)

DOI: 10.4324/9781003485346

Typeset in Times New Roman
by Taylor & Francis Books

For Preston

Contents

Acknowledgements

Many people and organizations supported me in the research, writing, and publication of this book. I want to first acknowledge two publications which permitted me to reprint my work.

First, the journal *Psychoanalytische Perspectieven* published my paper titled "The Ethics of Speech: Lacan, Francis, and the Real" in 2024 (Vol. 42, No. 1). This paper was originally presented on a panel on Lacan and religion at the Lacan: Clinic & Culture (2022) conference in Pittsburgh, PA. The three chapters in the first section of this book are a major expansion of the themes in this paper.

Second, *Integratus: Journal of the Catholic Psychotherapy Association* published my paper "'Making the Holy Obscene': A Thematic Analysis of Freudian Psychoanalysis in the Catholic Press" in 2024 (Vol. 2, No. 1). The section detailing Freud's essays on religion is reproduced in chapter one.

The John Martin Finlay poem "Two Poems for Oedipus" quoted in chapter nine is used with permission from Wiseblood Books.

The fifth chapter on Rahner and Lacan was first presented at a salon and two further discussions hosted by the Catholic Psychotherapy Association (2024). I thank them for the invitation and the feedback which contributed to strengthening the final version of the chapter.

The seventh chapter on priestly and psychoanalytic formation was originally presented at the Lacan Today (2024) conference in Ghent, Belgium on a panel with some of my favorite colleagues. I thank my colleagues and the audience for their feedback on that presentation.

My dear friend Hilary Zipperstein read drafts of almost every chapter and provided me with essential, critical perspectives to help me understand my own arguments and articulate them so eventual readers could understand them too. My colleagues Mason Judy and Nick Barkalow also reviewed chapters and provided their helpful insights.

I also need to acknowledge the support of Dr. Joy Schroeder, professor emerita of church history at Capital University, for writing a letter of recommendation on my behalf for access to the Vatican Archives.

The staff at the Archivio Apostolico Vaticano (Vatican Apostolic Archives) and the Archivio del Dicastero per la Dottrina della Fede (Archives of the Dicastery for the Doctrine of the Faith) were responsive, reliable, and patient with me. Without their assistance, I could not have written the sections on the history of censorship of psychoanalysis.

My Archbishop and his Executive Assistant were instrumental in helping me connect with officials at the Vatican. I am extremely grateful for such support at the diocesan level.

The personal faith experience which inspired this book is rooted in my faith community at Our Lady of the Lake Catholic Church. My priest, Father Tim Clark, welcomed me into the church and has provided me with ample spiritual direction and support. McKenzie Mauss facilitated my RCIA experience. Her passion, knowledge, and lived example of her faith was essential in my faith formation and decision to seek confirmation. In addition, all the members of my RCIA cohort, as well as the two cohorts I volunteered with later, all contributed to the insights and arguments in this book.

Each of the psychotherapists and psychoanalysts with whom I have worked as a patient and supervisee helped me grow and change into who I am today. This book reflects me as a work in progress.

I want to acknowledge the team at Routledge. My editor, Susannah Frearson, encouraged and supported me in writing my first book. Saloni Singhania facilitated all the necessary details to make publication possible. Laurence Fenton was the copyeditor and identified numerous ways to improve the manuscript and ensure accurate references. The final quality of the book is thanks to them.

Chair 13 at the bar of Long Bros. Fine & Rare Books was an orienting location from which to write on Friday afternoons. Surrounded by the works of esteemed writers and provided with ample fuel, I completed multiple chapters in that seat with the support of their staff.

Finally, I need to thank my parents. They initiated me into my Christian faith. They have lived their faith in service to many of our community's most vulnerable children, teenagers, and adults for decades. They taught me that my strengths, gifts, and privileges must be freely given for the needs of others.

Part I

History

Chapter 1

In the Beginning was Freud

Any dialogue between Catholicism and psychoanalysis must begin with Sigmund Freud (1856–1939). His identity as an esteemed neurologist, secular Jew, and pioneer psychoanalyst is well known. His theses on psychosexual development and the etiology and treatment of psychopathology along with critical commentaries on culture have been studied since their initial publications. Freud has never left print or conversation.

The purpose of this chapter is to review his relevant literature on religion and the responses his work generated in Catholicism. Freud was simultaneously critical and appreciative of the role of religion in the psychology of the individual and society. This history is explicated on a theoretical *and* personal level, for Freud is often misunderstood when the reader omits the personal level. This balanced reading is especially prudent for his work on religion.

The rest of this chapter examines the early history of this relationship through prominent figures who worked at this intersection. France took center stage, as Catholicism and psychoanalysis emerged intertwined following the Second World War. The life and work of Maryse Choisy is important to this history. Choisy was analyzed by Freud and later converted to Catholicism. She was close to Jacques Lacan and the French school of psychoanalysis. She was editor of the journal *Psyché*, which printed dialogue between psychoanalysis and religion. Many clergy and analysts joined her effort to sustain cooperative dialogue. Her life and work were a genealogical bridge from Freud to the Church.

Yet this adult convert saw her work censored by the *Suprema Sacra Congregatio Sancti Officii* (Supreme Sacred Congregation of the Holy Office, hereafter SSCSO) (1956a, 1956b) of the Vatican for reasons elaborated below. Father Agostino Gemelli wanted to sever this relationship between the Church and psychoanalysis. Gemelli, after whom the papal hospital in Rome is named, was a key influence in the speeches given by Pope Pius XII, who was the first Bishop of Rome to comment on psychoanalysis.

Pius XII criticized psychoanalysis within the wider context of *ressourcement* theology, which challenged the Neo-Scholastic theology that had been dominant in the Magisterium since the First Vatican Council. Unfortunately, suspicion and hostility, rather than trust and love, came to define this relationship.

DOI: 10.4324/9781003485346-2

Freud and Religion

Freud psychoanalyzed religious practices as obsessive actions (1959) and its doctrines as psychological illusions (1961). In his 1907 essay "Obsessive Actions and Religious Practices," he distinguished the similarities and differences between obsessional neurosis and its symptoms and religious "ceremonial" practices. Freud (1959) wrote that whereas the individual obsessional person has "variability" in symptoms compared to others, religious "ceremonial actions" are standardized. Whereas symptoms of obsessional neurosis are consciously meaningless, ceremonial actions are understood by the participants to have significant meaning. Furthermore, whereas obsessional neurotic individuals keep their actions as private as possible, ceremonial actions are completed in public (Freud, 1959, p. 118). And, while obsessional actions are "exclusively sexual in their origin," ceremonial actions in religion "spring from egoistic sources" (Freud, 1959, p. 126).

However, Freud (1959) argued a common developmental process is at work in both obsessional and ceremonial actions. First, the person experiences a sense of guilt, whether conscious or unconscious, driven by temptations with "contemporary provocation" (Freud, 1959, p. 122). There is both guilt for experiencing the desire and fear of the consequence of enacting the desire.

The Christian doctrine of original sin, for Freud, was akin to the individual obsessional neurotic's guilt: "The sense of guilt of obsessional neurotics finds its counterpart in the protestations of pious people that they know that at heart they are miserable sinners" (Freud, 1959, p. 122). Then, both obsessional and ceremonial actions function as "an action for defense or insurance, a protective measure" against the desire/instinct as well as the potential consequence (Freud, 1959, p. 122).

Yet Freud (1959, p. 123) argued that these defensive actions are not sustainable. Therefore "prohibitions come into play" as a kind of replacement for the action. A ceremonial action, for Freud, represents both the prohibition of acting on instinct and the instinct's permission. However, in both obsessional neurosis and religious practice, the "pleasure" the actions are meant to guard against becomes reproduced.

In religion, "complete backsliding into sin is more common among pious people than among neurotics," and this phenomenon leads to the next development, acts of penance (Freud, 1959, p. 124). In the end, Freud conceptualized "obsessional neurosis as a pathological counterpart of the formation of a religion" and concluded that there was a great deal of crossover between "neurosis as an individual religiosity and religion as a universal obsessional neurosis" (Freud, 1959, pp. 125–126).

Two decades later, in 1927, Freud published "The Future of an Illusion" (1961). Here he defined a belief as an illusion when a "wish fulfillment is a prominent factor in its motivation" and the belief is unverifiable in the strict notion of science familiar to Freud (1961, p. 56). Freud noted that illusions are not necessarily false (making them different from delusions) nor are illusions simply errors. He used Christopher Columbus's belief that he had traversed a new route to the Indies as an example of an illusion; Columbus *wished* for this discovery, his wish made his belief true, and there was (at the time) no way of verifying whether his belief was true (Freud, 1961, p. 55).

Freud (1961, p. 55) then applied his definition of illusion to religion. Religious ideas, "given out as teachings, are not precipitates of experience or end-results of thinking: they are illusions, fulfillment of the oldest, strongest and most urgent wishes of mankind." Freud postulated early humanity as "helpless" and in need of "protection" in much the same way as a child needs a parent.

That people believed in deities reflected their desire for protection. Freud cited theologians like Tertullian as evidence that religious practitioners saw their faith as outside the realm of reason. Therefore, "all of them are illusions and insusceptible to proof" (Freud, 1961, p. 57). Unsurprisingly, as Foschi et al. (2018, p. 3) argued, "Freud's publication of *'The Future of an Illusion'* in 1927 marked the Church's transition to a phase of open hostility toward psychoanalysis."

Despite this critical analysis, Freud's personal engagement with religious people was warm. The primary example of this warmth was his friendship and correspondence with the Protestant pastor Oskar Pfister (1873–1956). In Freud's correspondence with Pfister (Meng & Freud, 2023, p. 16), religion, rather than being a source of or defense against neurosis, was for Freud "sublimation in its most comfortable form." From Pfister, Freud learned "how extraordinarily helpful the psycho-analytic method might be in pastoral work," but because he saw himself as a "wicked pagan," such application was beyond his nature (Meng & Freud, 2023, p. 17).

Freud's analysis was focused on the theological teaching of the Church. He had not, until Pfister, considered pastoral work. Through this relationship, Freud learned that while the Magisterium's function is to teach, the pastor's function is to love. Freud personally experienced, and deeply appreciated, this pastoral love. Freud would later conclude, "The words 'secular pastoral worker' might well serve as a general formula for describing the function which the analyst, whether he is a doctor or a layman, has to perform in his relation to the public" (1964, pp. 255–256).

Pfister applied his initial understanding of psychoanalysis to Christian history.

> The Reformation was fundamentally nothing but an analysis of Catholic sexual repression, unfortunately a totally inadequate one, hence the anxiety neurosis of church orthodoxy and the concomitant phenomena – the witch trials, political absolutism, the social rigidity of the guild system, etc.
>
> (Meng & Freud, 2023, p. 18)

Where Freud analyzed standard religious practices as obsessional actions, Pfister widened the scope in his analysis of the Catholic Church's historical wrongdoing in facilitating persecution of heretics with its unquestionable authority. That Pfister saw the Reformation as inadequate to address Catholic repression is important. Protestants committed acts as egregious as the Church against which they protested.

Freud referred to Pfister as a "Man of God" and "too decent of a man," and regularly insisted Pfister submit his works for publication in the psychoanalytic publications of his time (Meng & Freud, 2023, pp. 29, 38). Freud told Pfister he valued "[his] enthusiasm, [his] integrity, and love of humanity, [his] courage and candour, [his] understanding and also – [his] optimism" (Meng & Freud, 2023, p. 61). Pfister was just as effusive of Freud, whom he referred to as a "noble Nathan" (an Old Testament prophet and advisor to King David). Pfister "quickly fell in love with [Freud's] humanitarian character" and described Freud's home as "the most agreeable place in the world" (Meng & Freud, 2023, pp. 90–91).

Freud wondered why he, a "godless Jew," discovered analysis given that the "predecessors in psychoanalysis" were "the Catholic fathers" (Meng & Freud, 2023, p. 21). Pfister, ever the pastor, did not accept Freud's often cynical self-assessments. He insisted on Freud's goodness rooted in the image of God. Pfister challenged Freud in this regard.

> In the first place you are no [religious] Jew, which to me, in view of my unbounded admiration for Amos, Isaiah, Jeremiah, and the author of Job and Ecclesiastes, is a matter of profound regret, and in the second place you are not godless, for he who lives in truth lives in God, and he who strives for the freeing of love "dwelleth in God" (First Epistle of John, iv, 16).
>
> (Meng & Freud, 2023, p. 63)

Pfister understood the most important connection between himself and Freud, and between Christianity and psychoanalysis, was the pursuit and embodiment of truth. This truth is deeply personal and is only understood when experienced interpersonally with an Other. Pfister ended this same letter with a provocative claim:

> If you raised to your consciousness and fully felt your place in the great design, which to me is as necessary as the synthesis of the notes is to a Beethoven symphony, I should say of you: *A better Christian there never* was.
>
> (Meng & Freud, 2023, p. 63, emphasis added)

Pfister interpreted Freud's religious character as unconscious but unmistakably present.

Freud recognized "the transference is indeed a cross" (Meng & Freud, 2023, p. 39), which suggests he suffered a sense of being forsaken by God.

Pfister recognized the necessary counterbalance that Freud's wife, children, and friends played with Freud's often pessimistic view of humanity. Without relationships, without love, Freud would have been unable to sustain the development of his healing method which continues to influence psychology to this day. As Pfister understood, despite all his protestations and cynicism, Freud loved humanity, especially the people whom society at large marginalized and judged from a perverse sense of superiority.

"A better Christian there never was" – such an introduction to Freud sounds absurd to modern ears. Though this statement came from a Protestant pastor, this perspective is crucial to understand how and why Freud's work, and psychoanalysis in general, is relevant to Catholics now. The primary argument of this book is that the world needs both Catholicism and psychoanalysis because of their insistence on pursuing the truth. Neither anthropology can conduct this pursuit alone. As demonstrated between Pfister and Freud, there must be an honest, loving relationship between the two to experience truth. For more information and analysis of this relationship, Domínguez-Moreno (2024) wrote an extensive commentary worth reading.

Maryse Choisy

In 1925, a 22-year-old French aristocratic woman named Maryse Choisy (1903–1979) traveled 1,500 kilometers to Wien IX, Berggasse 19, in Vienna to begin her psychoanalysis with Sigmund Freud. By this time, Freud was in his early seventies and famous. Nearly a quarter of a century after his publication of *The Interpretation of Dreams* (1900), his work had generated significant interest and controversy. Choisy (1963, p. 1) approached him with awe and literal breathlessness:

> Never did my heart beat for a lover as it did the day I walked up the Berggasse. Was that Vienna street really a steep climb? Or did it only appear so to me because I was at last going to see my God (at that time), who by some miracle had become accessible?

Choisy idealized the man. Once in the consulting room, she closely examined his "thin lips, his ascetic chin, his small gestures" (Choisy, 1963, p. 3). She searched for the truth of the man. Her expectations were shaken by reality. "Freud was rude. Yes, that bitter, misanthropic, utterly pessimistic outlook was Freud's business" (Choisy, 1963, p. 3). She confronted Freud the clinician. "My analysis started out with spirit, enthusiasm and speed. It went *too well*" (Choisy, 1963, p. 5, emphasis in original). In the third session, she shared a dream which Freud interpreted as revealing a family secret. Choisy was shocked and "indignant" (Choisy, 1963, p. 6). Her idealization turned to devaluation. And yet, upon her return home, she learned from her family that Freud was correct.

That Freud deduced this secret after only three sessions and not knowing her family overwhelmed Choisy. "He saw through me. I felt as transparent as glass. I was scared. I was so scared that I would go to great lengths to avoid analysts. It took me eight years to overcome my panic" (Choisy, 1963, p. 7). While Choisy avoided psychoanalysts, she continued her research and writing. Choisy's work crossed various genres, from existential journalism to sociological analysis to gender studies to mysticism and the occult.

Choisy published *Un mois chez les filles, reportage* in 1928. This book reported her experience going undercover in a brothel. She humanized the lives and work of female sex workers in Paris and shed light on the coercive practices of the men who ran the institutions. However, she wrote explicit descriptions of the sexual encounters she observed in the brothel, which seemed to distract critics from the intention of the text.

Choisy then published *Un mois chez les hommes, reportage* in 1929, another undercover report, this time within the all-male monastery at Mount Athose in Greece. She disguised herself as a man, complete with a fake penis, to live alongside the monks. Readers were again more entertained and disgusted by Choisy's incredible efforts to place herself in this environment than the lessons she drew from her observations.

Then in 1930 Choisy published *L'Amour dans les prisons, reportage.* Choisy did not attempt an undercover assignment in male prisons in France for this investigation but visited and spoke with incarcerated men about how prison affected their relationship to women and sex. Their loss of freedom at large often meant an unholy chastity.

What these texts shared, with much of her other work, other than their genre of investigatory reporting and sociological analysis, was Choisy's interest in people who lived on the margins of society: prostitutes, monks, and convicted criminals. While monks may not appreciate being included in this list, it is clear that they share a private, secluded life often inaccessible to the public. The public does not clamor for such access. Yet Choisy's books were best sellers at the time. *Un mois chez les filles* sold between 200,000–350,000 copies when it was in print. Choisy's interest in the isolated, distant, unknown lives of others was not far afield from psychoanalysis.

Dates in the literature vary, but in the 1930s, Choisy converted to Catholicism amidst her re-engagement with psychoanalysis (Cosnier, 2005, p. 290). For Choisy, personally and professionally, one anthropology required the other. The Dutch Jesuit priest and anthropologist Father Teilhard de Chardin was responsible for her conversion to Catholicism while her embrace of psychoanalysis was facilitated in part through her two analyses with Rene Laforgue (whom she idealized) and Maurice Bouvet (whom she devalued) (Ohayan, 2006, p. 325). Her panic subsided and she surrounded herself with psychoanalysts and priests.

Choisy recognized her dual commitment to Freud's legacy and the doctrine of her new Church was uncommon. She was an isolated member of a small community. With support from her like-minded friends and colleagues, particularly Laforgue, Choisy created and edited the journal *Psyché, Revue internationale de Psychanalyse et des Sciences de l'Homme* from 1946–1963. The journal represented one front in Choisy's larger project to have psychoanalysis officially recognized as legitimate theory and practice by the Catholic Church. She also sought to soften the historical hostility psychoanalysis brought to its perspective on religion.

Choisy (1951) outlined her mission in an article titled "Psychoanalysis and Catholicism," originally given as a paper at a conference for L'Institut Catholique de Pedagogie in Ghent, Belgium in 1949. She quoted from what Freud considered to be his "worst book," "The Future of an Illusion": "Nevertheless the defenders of religion have an equal right to use psychoanalysis in order to appreciate truly the affective importance of religious doctrine" (Choisy, 1951, p. 75). Choisy interpreted this remark as a "challenge" which gave her the idea to create *Psyché*. She argued her work was a legitimate extension of applied psychoanalysis permitted by Freud.

Choisy (1951, 79) identified three "difficulties" between Catholicism and Freudianism: "1. the Freudian theory of sexuality. 2. the question of determinism and freedom. 3. the unconscious feeling of guilt and the dogma of sin." Choisy expanded on these ideas one year after her talk in Ghent in her book *Psychanalyse et Catholicisme* (1950). To her list of difficulties above she added Freud's atheism and moral responsibility (Choisy, 1950, p. 16).

While laypeople may have been offended by Freud's criticisms of religion, clerical readers simply brushed them aside. Father Agostino Gemelli O.F.M., a friar, medical doctor, and psychologist (after whom the current papal hospital in Rome is named), recognized "Freud is far removed from the world of religion, and especially from the Catholic world, so that any conversation on this subject with him or with one of his faithful followers is out of the question" (1955, p. 11). This remark was not a call to suppression or avoidance but a logical deduction.

Given that Freud was untrained in matters of theology and history, Gemelli saw it as unfair and/or unfruitful to engage with Freud on those topics. Instead, Gemelli, a trained psychologist, sought to engage Freud on psychological matters where they shared some level of education, competence, and practice. Gemelli vehemently disagreed with Freud, but he respected Freud's training and experience and wanted his criticisms to be grounded in a common framework.

Choisy argued Freud's conclusions about religion were not a definitive explanation of religious belief and practice. While Freud postulated religion as a product of the psychosexual development for the individual and culture, Choisy (1951, p. 25) argued, "God may have traced this biopsychological path to Love...Grace takes natural paths." Choisy paralleled the argument in favor of the theory of evolution. Psychoanalysis no more disputed humanity's origin in God than did evolution, given that God uses both processes to the good of His creation.

Whenever psychoanalysis, as Choisy understood it, came into conflict with Catholic theology, she deferred to the doctrine of the Magisterium. After her conversion, and her writing becoming more focused on religion, the Church familiarized itself with her past work.

Her decision in 1954 to pull *Un mois chez les filles* from the market was due to pressure from the SSCSO in Vatican City. In a report prepared by the SSCSO about her later books, Father Udalricus Beste O.S.B. noted Choisy had "already [been] condemned by the Holy Office two years ago, and the withdrawal of her work cost her 200,000 francs" (1956b, p. 2). Choisy was willing to sacrifice personal finances as well as psychoanalytic theory to please the Vatican.

However, in Choisy's attempt to bridge the gap between psychoanalysis and Catholicism, she relented on the existence of morality in psychoanalysis. "Psychoanalysis, like any science, is neither moral nor immoral" (Choisy, 1951, p. 27). While it is true that the psychoanalyst does not take a moral stance regarding the patient's conduct in the session, it is not accurate that morality is absent from psychoanalytic theory. The attempt to remove morality from psychoanalysis was Choisy's way of making psychoanalysis more palatable to Catholic readers and leaders.

This strategy was not successful. On January 21, 1952, consultors for the SSCSO unanimously recommended *Psychoanalysis and Catholicism* be "withdrawn from sale" and, if that were not done, "an article should be published in *L'Osservatore Romano,* in which the book should be rejected" (1956a, p. 3). The Holy Office threatened to publicly condemn the book in its official newspaper unless Choisy censored her work. Thus, two of Choisy's books were removed from the market due to the influence of the Vatican.

This strategy of behind-the-scenes censorship and public condemnation if necessary was common for the Holy Office (see chapter four). The consultors concluded, "*Quod psychoanalysim, silendum*" (SSCSO, 1956a, p. 3). As for psychoanalysis, it should be kept quiet. Nine days later, Pope Pius XII approved the decree.

A few months later, from April 7–13, 1953, the Catholic Congress of Psychotherapy and Psychology was held in Rome. The President of this group was Father Gemelli. Maryse Choisy was the General Secretary. Choisy was scheduled to present a report to the group, as was Father Marc Oraison (another target of Church censorship). Both reports were removed from the schedule at the direct request of the Holy Office (SSCSO, 1956a, p. 4).

Near the conclusion of the conference, on April 11, 1953, Pope Pius XII provided a speech titled "On Psychotherapy and Religion" in which he argued psychology and psychoanalysis need to be practiced within the confines of Catholic moral teaching. This speech is outlined below.

Choisy published two more texts after her conversion and around the time of this conference – *Le scandale de l'amour* (The Scandal of Love, 1954) and *Problèmes sexuels de l'adolescence* (Sexual Problems of Adolescence, 1954).

These were reviewed by the Holy Office (SSCSO, 1956a). The report included "votes" by Father Phillipe of the Trinity, O.C.D. and Canon Joseph Geraud of St. Sulpice. These reviewers were no strangers to psychoanalysis.

The two texts were understood to continue Choisy's commitment to "Freudian principles and statements on a moral level (about sex) which are unacceptable" (SSCSO, 1956a, p. 5). Phillipe and Geraud provided independent analyses of both texts and concluded with a vote as to whether the texts should be censored and placed on the *Index Librorum Prohibitorum* (Index of Prohibited Books).

Phillipe, at the beginning of his analysis of *Sexual Problems of Adolescence*, quoted Choisy regarding the definition of sexual. Choisy herself referenced Freud. "From the beginning," wrote Choisy, "I warned that what Freud meant by sexuality encompassed the entire capacity of man to love and hate" (SSCSO, 1956a, p. 5). This expansive definition of sexuality, entirely correct in its Freudian application, was provided without comment from Phillipe. Yet it is this radical idea which is at the heart of Freudian theory.

The report began with significant praise for Choisy.

> The book is very well written, occasionally full of humor and wit; the intentions are excellent, and the general thrust of the presentation seems very good to me: about life, common sense, and a genuine concern for morality. Freudian themes are found, but, in my opinion, in their relevance to Christian thought (the discussion remains open, of course).
> (SSCSO, 1956a, p. 6)

However, Phillipe shared several concerns. He questioned Choisy's argument that in education, the ovary should be taught as objectively as the gallbladder or spleen. Phillipe questioned, "With the same level of detail? And would it depend on the age, in which class?" (SSCSO, 1956a, p. 6). One senses a tension for Phillipe; at one level he agrees to a generally scientific approach to the study and teaching of the body but is wary of explicit details which might violate Catholic moral standards and potentially incite arousal in students learning about certain body parts.

On masturbation, Choisy provocatively argued, "Guilt is more dangerous for the adolescent's wellbeing than masturbation" (SSCSO, 1956a, p. 6). Phillippe asked, "What kind of guilt is this?" (SSCSO, 1956a, p. 6). Were it psychopathological guilt, he would agree. If it were moral guilt, he would not agree. This distinction between types of guilt is important. What is nonpathological guilt? And at what point does it become pathological? And how does one address each of them in turn? Does treatment for psychopathological guilt restore a healthy moral guilt?

Yet the implication that the moral dimension can be neatly separated from the psychological dimension, or one subsumed under the other, often does not reflect the lived experience of many people experiencing guilt.

Another important question which Phillipe did not raise is: what kind of wellbeing is this? Physiological? Psychological? Spiritual? And what designates wellbeing? The absence of suffering? The presence of contentment? All these questions complicate a simple, rigid doctrinal stance against the behavior of masturbation, and indeed any sexual act.

Phillipe was also attentive to Choisy's discussion of the development of sexual desire. "To sublimate," Choisy argued, "one must initially have a force" (SSCSO, 1956a, p. 7). Choisy did not argue for complete unrestraint for sexual desire and activity, hence her reference to sublimation. Choisy was concerned that excessive suppression and punishment of all sexual activity in adolescence would put out the pilot light of desire in general, which would produce an "inhibited being" unable to participate in social or spiritual life.

In the end, despite Phillipe's conclusion that "the work as a whole is good," he recommended Choisy be warned about its doctrinal errors, withdraw the current edition from sale, and revise and correct it before seeking republication (SSCSO, 1956a, p. 8). Interestingly, Phillipe did not recommend the book be placed on the Index, as "for these kinds of books, the Index represents excellent publicity" (SSCSO, 1956a, p. 9). Censorship of the text would prompt the desire to read it! Prohibition prompts desire, an ironically Freudian idea.

Geraud objectively outlined each of the chapters without comment before he offered his value judgment of the text. He noted Choisy applied Freud's principles and methods to the problems of adolescence. On this point, he did not object to a scientific approach to a modern problem. Though he disagreed with Freudian theory, he did not dispute the right of an author to present a philosophical system.

His issue was Choisy's claim to "speak as a Christian to Christian women" and the way in which she presented Freudian theory as "undisputed scientific truth" (SSCSO, 1956a, p. 11). He was concerned with the praise the work received and the recommendations to priests and nuns to read it. Geraud had "serious reservations" about the text given that Choisy, from his perspective, downplayed concerns with sexual behaviors like masturbation and premarital sex which the Church explicitly prohibited (SSCSO, 1956a, p. 12). However, he did not state a conclusion or recommendation as to what should be the fate of the text. This reticence may have been due to the fact the book was not officially sanctioned by church authorities, like *The Scandal of Love.*

Despite a respectable goal, *The Scandal of Love* was a "painful and tedious read" for Geraud (SSCSO, 1956a, p. 36). He cited "dangerous or erroneous" passages which represented his core criticisms (SSCSO, 1956a, p. 37). First, Choisy offered a "purely Freudian interpretation of Redemption" (SSCSO, 1956a, p. 37). Choisy compared the story and aim of Redemption to the process of initiating and resolving transference with the psychoanalyst and the intrapsychic process of sublimation. Geraud thought such an interpretation introduced determinism into Redemption (contrary to the agency which theology insists each person possesses). Here, determinism is attributed to psychoanalytic theory in a way which misunderstood Freud's intent.

Second, Geraud argued Choisy reduced chastity "to a kind of magic" (SSCSO, 1956a, p. 37) due to her many references to ancient cultures and mythologies. But Geraud, though he quoted passages, seemed to miss the feminism at the core of Choisy's critique and function of chastity. "It wasn't woman who invented it," noted Choisy (SSCSO, 1956a, p. 37). She pointed to the power dynamic chastity has been designed in part to address. By remaining chaste, a man "proves to himself that he can do without woman, her heart, her abyss, and her love" (SSCSO, 1956a, p. 38). Choisy did not claim this is the sole meaning and function of chastity but given her extensive ethnological research into how people relate to sex, she saw power as an important factor.

Third, Geraud criticized Choisy's commentary on "passionate love" (SSCSO, 1956a, pp. 37–38). He seemed offended by the explicit language Choisy used in detailing how women relate to their bodies in sexual activity. She focused on how women begin with ignorance and, without other women to guide them in understanding their bodies, explore and discover passion. Despite his offense, Geraud quoted without commentary several passages of explicit sexual activity. Perhaps he thought the passages would speak for themselves in terms of their inappropriateness for publication.

In the end, Geraud argued Choisy's text was "truly a bad book" (SSCSO, 1956a, p. 43). He felt strongly that it would be "dangerous to let such a book slip by and allow it to be spread" (SSCSO, 1956a, p. 44). Geraud was aware, like Phillipe, that a public denouncement would potentially increase the number of readers. He instead favored a "discreet" solution, the withdrawal of the book from sale and publication of a revised edition at a later date (SSCSO, 1956a, p. 44). Given that Geraud took issue with each of the primary themes of the text, it is unclear what revisions would have satisfied him.

Phillipe did not agree with Geraud's vehement criticisms of the text. He disagreed with Geraud's characterization of Choisy as clearly Freudian. Phillipe argued, "If she draws inspiration from Freud from a psychological perspective (and this is legitimate; see the thesis of the excellent Thomist R. Dalbiez, *The Psychoanalytic Method and the Freudian Doctrine*), she positively rejects Freud's erroneous metaphysical and moral positions" (SSCSO, 1956a, p. 14).

Phillipe saw no intent from her to scandalize readers or lead people to commit immoral acts. He respected the scientific genre of the work and assessed it on its own terms. He took issue with some of the language and terms Choisy used and exaggerations she made about theological matters. While Phillipe seemed to take some interest in the text, he did not seem to worry much about its influence.

> Personally, it would not seem appropriate to me to place the book on the Index, nor to withdraw it from sale...I believe that M. Choisy should not be given more importance than she deserves. M. Choisy is in decline. At the International Catholic Congress of Psychotherapy and Clinical Psychology in Ettal (September 4–10, 1955), I was able to observe that she was no longer considered an authority, if she ever had been (which is doubtful).
>
> (SSCSO, 1956a, p. 24)

Choisy was therefore seen as a sincere Catholic earnest in her intention to integrate her faith and work. Church officials spent considerable ink when they investigated her texts. Some officials valued her work. Others painted her work, like psychoanalysis in general, as unscientific, immoral, and dangerous. Father Beste (SSCSO, 1956b, p. 4) concluded, "poison is produced by reading" her work. In the end, she was seen as irrelevant to the profession and Church. Psychoanalysis as a whole, however, remained top of mind for the Church as the decade progressed.

Pius XII and Psychoanalysis

Pope Pius XII gave speeches in 1952 and 1953 which outlined official papal limitations on psychoanalytic theory and practice. The first speech was an address which concluded the First International Congress on the Histopathology of the Nervous System titled *The Moral Limits of Medical Research and Treatment* in 1952. Pius XII claimed a broad deontological framework within which practitioners and researchers were permitted to operate, according to his teaching and the moral authority of the Church.

Pius XII (1952, para. 5) identified three "principles" which must be contemplated to justify a medical intervention: the interests of medical science, the interests of the individual patient to be treated, and the interests of the community. These interests constitute both the moral justification for medical research and treatment and its moral limitations.

First, the interest of medical science is an interest in the advancement of knowledge. As Pius XII (1952, para. 7) argued, "knowledge as such and the full understanding of any truth raise no moral objection." However, where the pursuit of knowledge in medicine is not inherently immoral, it is also not inherently moral. Pius XII continued:

> But this does not mean that all methods, or any single method, arrived at by scientific and technical research offers every moral guarantee. Nor, moreover, does it mean that every method becomes licit because it increases and deepens our knowledge.
>
> (1952, para. 8)

Pius XII argued that "science is not the highest value" and therefore "must be inserted in the order of values" taught by the Church.

Second, the interest of the patient involves informed consent. Here Pius XII again argued against an absolute value assigned to this interest, stating (1952, para. 12), "the decisive point is the moral licitness of the right a patient has to dispose of himself." As science is not the highest value, neither is human will.

The patient "is not absolute master of himself, of his body or of his soul. He cannot, therefore, freely dispose of himself as he pleases" (Pius XII, 1952, para. 13). The patient's desire and approval of treatment is not enough to justify the moral nature of the treatment because people exist within a moral hierarchy where God – and His Magisterium – hold final authority.

Pius XII (1952, para. 16) then spoke about psychoanalysis:

> In order to rid himself of repressions, inhibitions or psychic complexes man is not free to arouse in himself for therapeutic purposes each and every appetite of a sexual order which is being excited or has been excited in his being, appetites whose impure waves flood his unconscious or subconscious mind.

Pius XII disapproved of open-ended exploration of the unconscious for fear that doing so would promote unrestricted sexual desires and activities. On the one hand, Pius XII practically repeated Freud's famous dictum that ego is not the master in its own house. Yet Pius XII went further: ego may not be the master of its house, but God should be, and by transitive property, the Pope. He clearly recognized the validity of psychoanalytic concepts/phenomena but strongly opposed clinical practice which may disturb "underlying appetites."

Instead, Pius XII (1952, para. 17) argued psychotherapy should focus on the conscious mind: "Where instincts are concerned it would be better to pay more attention to indirect treatment and to the action of the conscious psyche on the whole of imaginative and affective activity."

Pius XII was highly invested in sustaining the defenses which hold back unconscious impulses and desires. As Pius XII (1952, para. 39) stated:

> The great moral demands force the impetuous flow of human thought and will to flow, like water from the mountains, into certain channels. They contain the flow to increase its efficiency and usefulness. They dam it so that it does not overflow and cause ravages that can never be compensated for by the special good it seeks.

The cost of Freudian psychoanalysis was greater than the benefit. Morality does not simply function as a "brake" on the speed of scientific advancement, but shapes and contours such progress into something more "beautiful" (Pius XII, 1952, para. 39). Without morality, psychoanalysis risks this beauty.

Finally, the interest of the community involved the subordination of the individual to the common good. Pius XII argued here against the idea that government permission for a doctor to perform an intervention or experiment provides moral justification for doing so. He used Nazi Germany as an example of how such an arrangement can violate moral law. Pius XII (1952, para. 29) argued the opposite principle, that "man is not finally ordered to usefulness to society. On the contrary, the community exists for man," echoing vaguely anti-communist sentiments.

One year later, Pius XII spoke to the large gathering of psychotherapists and psychologists headed by Gemelli and Choisy at the Fifth International Congress on Psychotherapy and Clinical Psychology. He sought to remind them of their place and role as being subject to this larger ethical/theological framework, "the fundamental attitude which is imposed upon the Christian psychologist and psychotherapeutist" (Pius XII, 1953, para. 4).

Through reason and fate, Pius XII (1953, para. 5) stated:

> Psychotherapy and clinical psychology must always consider man 1. as a psychic unit and totality 2. as a structured unit in itself 3. as a social unit, and 4. as a transcendent unit, that is to say, in man's tending towards God.

In the conceptualization of man as a psychic unit and totality, Pius XII argued the soul is the core of human existential experience. "From it, ultimately, flows all the vital activity of man. In it are rooted all the psychic dynamisms with their own proper structure and their organic law" (Pius XII, 1953, para. 7). Such a statement appeared to counter the primacy psychoanalysis places on the unconscious as the seat of human desire and activity.

Where psychoanalysts might ascribe an unwanted behavior to a repressed desire, and therefore explore its unconscious determinants, Pius XII advocated for a deeper, theological level to human experience. "To deprive the soul of its central place would be to deny an ontological and psychic reality" (Pius XII, 1953, para. 8). This deprivation of the soul is, in essence, to deny human freedom to act in accordance with his will, and the will of God. Pius XII argued against the conception of unconscious instincts being the core motivator of human behavior.

The second principle, man as a structured unit, was a continuation of Pius XII's remarks in 1952 which detailed a hierarchy of academic and clinical disciplines. Psychology belongs within the realm of theology and ontology, not the other way around. Pius XII argued the theory of the unconscious and the clinical implications of such theory must fit within the larger metaphysical framework of Christian theology and morality.

Finally, the third principle, man as social unit, which Pius XII described as "the study of the psychic in its social aspects, in itself and in its roots" (1953, para. 18). Social psychological research and treatment also needed to be limited on moral grounds. Pius XII identified two errors which can occur in this work.

First, "error by defect" (Pius XII, 1953, para. 20). Pius XII here took issue with the conceptualization of psychological issues occurring due to the "inhibition of the ego." Not all inhibition should be seen as pathological; indeed, morality demands some degree of inhibition of sexual impulses. Therefore, psychotherapy and psychoanalysis must leave these inhibitions in place. Again, Pius XII promoted conscious-driven interventions, for example, (limited) sexual education to address psychological issues with sexuality.

Second, "error by excess" (Pius XII, 1953, para. 25). Pius XII argued against, on the one hand, the emphasis on altruism, and on the other hand, emphasis on defensive mechanisms, that different schools of psychology and psychoanalysis have attributed to the purpose of the ego. The ego is not something which should be indiscriminately deconstructed in the pursuit of repressed knowledge or therapeutic cure.

Pius XII used natural philosophy to affirm the need for some level of secrecy, of repression, in the patient, when he stated (1953, para. 27):

> It is not at all excluded that a fact or knowledge which is secret and repressed in the subconscious provokes serious psychic conflicts. If psychoanalysis discloses the cause of this trouble, it will want, according to its principle, to draw out entirely this unconscious element and make it conscious in order to remove the obstacle. But there are secrets which must on no account be divulged, even to a doctor, even in spite of grave personal inconveniences.

Pius XII argued that simply because a fact or piece of knowledge has been subject to repression does not mean it inevitably produces psychic conflict. Therefore, there is no need for the clinician and patient to make the unconscious conscious. Pius XII instead argued that it would be better for society if those repressions remained intact. In Pius XII's perspective, without Catholic morality, psychoanalysis was dangerous to the individual and society.

The final principle is "man as a transcendent unit, tending towards God" (Pius XII, 1953). Here, Pius XII addressed the attempt, beginning with Freud, of an analysis of religious belief and practice. He stated (1953, para. 32):

> We should certainly not find fault with depth psychology if it deals with the psychic aspect of religious phenomena and endeavors to analyze and reduce it to a scientific system, even if this research is new and if its terminology is not found in the past.

The attempt at developing a conceptualization as to how and why people engage with religion on a psychological level can provide valuable knowledge to the Church. But Pius XII stressed the need for reciprocity in this regard. If psychoanalysis is permitted to analyze religious belief, the Church must also have the permission to offer its own conceptualization and strategies for understanding and responding to psychological suffering.

To this end, Pius XII focused on the phenomenon of guilt as the Church and psychoanalysis both address it. While psychoanalysis can explore the psychic determinants of this feeling, Pius XII (1953, para. 36) argued, "it is certain that no purely psychological treatment will cure a genuine sense of guilt." There remains a need for absolution of the fault which prompted the guilt. Pius XII placed theology as the larger context within which psychology is permitted to operate.

Conclusion

Religion was, for Freud, one cultural phenomenon among many which illustrated the truth of the theoretical insights he learned from his psychoanalytic clinical practice. Freud in his writing accused Christianity of being an illusive crutch which offered nothing more than communal experience of obsessional neurosis. Yet in his personal relationships and his reflections on his work, he understood his practice as a pastoral vocation which accompanied people in their suffering without judgment or agenda. Freud never came close to experiencing personal religious belief. Yet the way in which he cared for people was undeniably Christ-like.

Maryse Choisy, one of the only people recorded as having been analyzed by Freud and then converted to Catholicism, recognized this tension. She attempted to reconcile the conflict which emerged between Catholicism and psychoanalysis through compromise. Through this work she intersected with some of the greatest minds of her day: Teilhard de Chardin, Rene Laforgue, Agostino Gemelli, and Jacques Lacan. Despite her effort and connections, she was unsuccessful in achieving papal approval of psychoanalysis. Her past, her gender, her personality, and her provocative writing were investigated, mocked, and dismissed. This failure came at great personal and financial cost. To risk hyperbole, Maryse Choisy was a martyr.

Pope Pius XII was the first pope to directly address psychoanalysis. While he recognized its validity in the same scope as general scientific research and practice, he did not accept its core claim of the existence and influence of the unconscious. All psychoanalytic theory and practice needed to constrain itself within the moral limits and responsibilities of Catholic Christianity as dictated by the Vatican. His criticism of psychoanalysis needs to be seen within the broader context of his suspicion of modernism within his Neo-Scholastic framework. With the passing of Pius XII and the election of John XXIII, the Church shifted into a more cooperative engagement with the modern world.

References

Choisy, M. (1950). *Psychanalyse et Catholicisme.* L'Arche Collection Commentaries. L'Arche.

Choisy, M. (1951). Psychoanalysis and Catholicism. (J.E. Cuneen, Trans.). *CrossCurrents,* 1(3): 75–90.

Choisy, M. (1963). *Sigmund Freud: A new appraisal.* Citadel Press.

Cosnier, J. (2005). Choisy, Maryse (1903–1979). In A. de Mijolla (Ed.), *International dictionary of psychoanalysis*, Volume 1, A–F (pp. 289–290). Macmillan Reference USA.

Domínguez-Moreno, C. (2024). *Sigmund Freud and Oskar Pfister on religion: The beginning of an endless dialogue.* (F. Montero, Trans.). Routledge. (Original work published 2000)

Foschi, R., Innamorati, M., & Taradel, R. (2018). "A disease of our time": The Catholic Church's condemnation and absolution of psychoanalysis (1924-1975). *Journal of the History of the Behavioral Sciences*, 54(2): 85–100. doi:10.1002/jhbs.21894

Freud, S. (1959). Obsessive actions and religious practices. In J. Strachey (Ed. & Trans.), *The standard edition of the complete psychological works of Sigmund Freud*, Vol. 9 (pp. 115–127). Hogarth Press. (Original work published 1907)

Freud, S. (1961). The future of an illusion. In J. Strachey (Ed. & Trans.), *The standard edition of the complete psychological works of Sigmund Freud*, Vol. 21 (pp. 1–56). Hogarth Press. (Original work published 1927)

Freud, S. (1964). The question of lay analysis. In J. Strachey (Ed. & Trans.), *The standard edition of the complete psychological works of Sigmund Freud*, Vol. 20: (pp. 179–258). Hogarth Press. (Original work published 1926)

Gemelli, A. (1955). *Psychoanalysis today.* P.J. Kennedy & Sons.

Lacan, J. (2013). *The triumph of religion preceded by discourse to Catholics.* (B. Fink, Trans.). Polity Press. (Original work published 2005)

Meng, H. & Freud, E. (2023). *Psychoanalysis and faith: The letters of Sigmund Freud and Oskar Pfister.* (E. Mosbacher, Trans.). Lushena Books.

Ohayan, A. (2006). *Psychologie et psychanalyse en France: L'impossible rencontre (1919–1969)*. La Découverte.

Pius XII. (1952). *Address to the participants in the first international congress on histopathology of the nervous system.* https://www.papalencyclicals.net/pius12/p12psych.htm.

Pius XII. (1953). *Speech by Pope Pius XII to participants in the international congress of psychotherapy and clinical psychology.* https://www.papalencyclicals.net/pius12/p12psyre.htm.

Suprema Sacra Congregatio Sancti Officii (SSCSO). (1956a). *Parigi. Dr Maryse Choisy: Relazione della cancelleria.* Prot. Num. 76/55/i; cfr. Num. 287/51. Archivio del Dicastero per la Dottrina della Fede. Vatican City.

Suprema Sacra Congregatio Sancti Officii (SSCSO). (1956b). *Parisien. Maryse Choisy: Correctio et eventualis reeditio operum: Problemes sexuels de l'adolescence, Le scanadale de l'amour.* Prot. Num. 76/55. Archivio del Dicastero per la Dottrina della Fede. Vatican City.

Chapter 2

Leuven's Legacy of Dialogue

From Mercier to Lacan

Pope Francis spoke to professors at the Catholic University of Leuven on the occasion of the 600th anniversary of its founding in September 2024. Pope Francis encouraged their broad, multidisciplinary pursuit of knowledge: "I would now like to extend a simple invitation to each of you: *expand the boundaries of knowledge!* Rather than multiplying concepts and theories, make academic and cultural formation a critical space that both understands and speaks about life" (2024, para. 3, emphasis in original).

Pope Francis affirmed the institution's connection to the papal bull of Pope Martin V through which he founded what is now known as the *Old* University of Leuven in 1425. Though the institutional history is complex due to nation state boundary changes, academic closures, reopenings, and splits, Pope Francis was proud to recognize the longstanding existence of Catholic education in the region. Pope Francis encouraged his audience to use knowledge as a means of understanding and speaking about life.

Psychoanalysis in Leuven

Though Pope Francis did not mention psychoanalysis in his address, the discipline has a long history in Leuven. Its history began about 500 years after the founding of the university, when Pope Leo XIII sought to revive the philosophical study of the work of Thomas Aquinas. A chair of Thomistic philosophy was created at Leuven and the man hired for the role was the future Cardinal Désiré Felicien François Joseph Mercier (1851–1926). Mercier was an alumnus of the university, having earned his licentiate in theology in 1877 and doctorate in philosophy and theology in 1882. Pope Leo XIII directly approved his hire and kept himself apprised of Mercier's work at the university.

Mercier felt strongly that philosophy must take account of modern science. As Misiak and Staudt (1954, p. 40) argued, Mercier sought "to integrate the truth of the old with the truth of the new." The discipline he first sought to understand and integrate was scientific psychology. The clinician and institution he sought for education was in Paris: Jean-Martin Charcot at the Salpêtriére Hospital. Mercier entered France during a particularly anticlerical

DOI: 10.4324/9781003485346-3

period. "Accordingly, he dressed as a layman" (Brown, 1927, p. 463) and "replaced his cassock with ordinary clothes and grew a beard" to study without the bias about his vocation (Misiak & Staudt, 1954, p. 41). Mercier fully committed to his mission.

Charcot should sound familiar to students of psychoanalysis because Charcot had another future famous student around the same time: Sigmund Freud. The exact timeline is unclear, but it appears Mercier visited Charcot for a brief period in 1882. At that time, Freud graduated from the University of Vienna and would arrive in Paris to study with Charcot in 1885. While this connection reflects the profound influence of Charcot on the trajectory of psychology, this shared education and training in Paris also demonstrates that both Catholicism and psychoanalysis have a historical commitment to learn and apply the latest knowledge in the field.

Mercier and Freud took different paths after they left Charcot. Mercier followed in the footsteps of Wilhelm Wundt into scientific and experimental psychology while Freud chartered his own trail into psychoanalysis. Three years prior to Freud's publication of *The Interpretation of Dreams* (1900), Mercier published *Les origines de la psychologie contemporaine* (The Origins of Contemporary Psychology, 1897). If Freud is the father of secular psychoanalysis, Mercier is the father of modern Catholic psychology.

Mercier criticized psychology for its philosophical foundation in Descartes. "The extreme dualism of the Cartesian psychology has become the original sin of contemporary psychology, for it set up an opposition between the soul, an unextended substance, and the body, an extended substance, possessing only mechanical motion" (Misiak & Staudt, 1954, p. 45). Mercier was opposed to the reduction of the human experience to biological and psychological fragments. He affirmed the necessity of metaphysics to psychology. That he understood original sin as the instantiation and experience of conflict, rather than a discrete behavior, is an insight carried forward in chapter five in this book.

While Freud and Mercier pursued different realms of study, and do not appear to have ever engaged the other's work, they recognized the fundamental connection between the mind and the body. This shared recognition is relevant today for Catholicism and psychoanalysis, as many modern psychological methods continue this dualism through similarly reductive interventions focused on training behaviors or balancing emotions.

While the unconscious and the soul are not the same, they share the essential truth about the unity of the person. Recognition of this unity is often neglected by psychoanalysts whose focus are the fragmented and conflicted parts of the person. Yet Catholicism sometimes moves too quickly to judge and absolve these conflicts, pursuing balance and peace at the cost of truth.

In 1923, just three years before the passing of Mercier, an American student at Leuven graduated with his doctorate in philosophy. His dissertation was bestowed with the Cardinal Mercier Prize for International Philosophy. This man became the Archbishop of New York, Fulton J. Sheen (1895–1979).

Sheen (1980, p. 25) thought he needed to learn two things, "first, what the modern world is thinking about; second, how to answer the errors of modern philosophy in light of the philosophy of St. Thomas." His advisor at the time told him, "You will never get it here, but you will get it at the University of Louvain in Belgium." Sheen began his studies in Leuven in September 1921.

Little is known about the curriculum in psychology he studied at Leuven, but Sheen carried forward an interest in the psychology of religion, in particular the psychology of conversion (1980, p. 134). Sheen insisted Catholic theology subsumed psychology within its metaphysics. "The psychological approach offers us no difficulty," Sheen (1949, p. 7) argued, "for Christian theology is, in a certain sense, a psychology, since its primary interest is the soul, the most precious of things."

Rather than see psychology and theology as partners in pursuing the truth of person, Sheen argued psychoanalysis was a product of a world which had disavowed God. Whereas man historically understood himself to live across a "three-dimensional universe" made up of Heaven above him, Earth with him, and Hell below him, without a belief in and relationship to God, man created three new dimensions "within his own mind" (Sheen, 1949, p. 3). Sheen argued:

> Above his *ego*, his conscious level, he discovers, in the place of heaven, an inexorable tyrant whom he calls the *super-ego*. Below his consciousness, in place of hell, he substitutes a hidden world of instincts and urges, primitive longings and biological needs, which he calls the *id*.
>
> (1949. p. 3, emphasis in original)

Sheen (1949, p. 11) taught psychopathology was estrangement from God: "Once the hub of the wheel, which is God, is lost, the spokes, which are men, fall apart." Sheen did not dispute the phenomenon of intrapsychic conflict. Indeed, psychology's explanation of this conflict could be useful.

> It may very well be that the new apologetic to the modern soul will start with the contributions of modern psychology on the subject of conflict, that it will be a kind of preface to the tract, *De peccato originali*, which is relatively the most important treatise on theology for the modern mind.
>
> (Sheen, 1949, p. 36)

That text, abbreviated DPO, was written by Hadriaan Beverland in 1679. Beverland was a Dutch humanist scholar who argued sex was the original sin in Genesis (Baines, 2025). That psychology would be but a preface to a humanist (but non-Christian) text demonstrated the limited utility Sheen (1949, p. 37) saw in the discipline, when he stated the "psychological is a superficial manifestation" of an ontological, universal conflict rooted in human nature. Sheen, though he may not have intended it, put sex at the center of that conflict.

For Sheen (1949, p. 46), a psychologist is but a bit player in the grand scheme of the universe: "A psychiatrist, a doctor, and a teacher may be able to relieve certain superficial complexes and conflicts, but no one is able to remove the basic cause of all complexes except God." Why work with a psychoanalyst to relieve a superficial complex when one could work with a priest and through his acting *in persona Christi*, receive the grace which removes the root cause of all complexes? The obvious answer, unaddressed by Sheen, is that millions of devoted Catholics continue to struggle with personal conflict despite their baptism, confirmation, and participation in the other sacraments. He did not acknowledge or explain this contradiction.

Bishop Sheen broadcasted a popular television program titled *Life is Worth Living* (1952–1957) which reached at its peak at over 30,000,000 viewers (Smith, 1997; Dennis, 2020). It is safe to say that no single psychoanalyst has ever had the reach to promote their practice as widely as Sheen did with his criticism. At least two episodes featured his critiques of psychoanalysis.

In an episode titled "Psychoanalytic Couch," Sheen contrasted two couches. First, the modern psychoanalytic couch pioneered by Freud. The person on this couch is the patient. The patient is passive, "he took his medicine lying down" (Connelly, 1956). On this couch, there is "no guilt…one never does anything wrong. One may have a complex, but one has never committed a sin." Sheen taught the psychoanalytic process made the person essentially disappear, body and soul, from their own life, to be filled by the interpretations of the analyst.

The second couch is the sort used in the ancient triclinium in Rome, a dining room where men would lay sideways and face each other as they ate and spoke. Sheen referred to the Gospel story when Jesus dined in the home of Simon the Pharisee. During the dinner, Jesus was the person on the couch. A woman approached his feet and began to weep. Ashamed, according to Sheen, she used her hair to wipe the tears and then used oil to anoint his feet. "It was guilt in her soul," said Sheen, "she had a sense of sin" (Connelly, 1956).

The following year, Sheen again addressed psychoanalysis in an episode titled "How to Psychoanalyze Yourself." "Anybody who goes to a psychoanalyst ought to have his head examined," Sheen said, to laughter from the audience (Connelly, 1957). Sheen wanted to argue what makes someone normal and what makes one abnormal, though not to a pathological degree. Sheen believed in the theory of mental illness but that it should be treated by medical doctors who specialized in psychiatry, not psychologists.

Sheen argued normal people have "purpose" and "meaning" in their life (Connelly, 1957). "Man must decide on that before he decides anything else." Sheen taught that the "normal goal" of human beings is happiness, truth, and love, all ultimately found in God. The abnormal man makes a "misplaced infinite." In other words, the abnormal person takes a material item for God. The normal person is also a person of reason whereas the abnormal person is driven by instincts and impulses and believes himself to be under the control of his subconscious mind. A normal man, with his purpose in mind, uses his reason and will to consciously pursue his goal.

Sheen used the metaphor of a captain of a ship directing the crew towards their final destination. An abnormal man has repressed his reason and will like an overturned ship and is submerged in the waters of the subconscious. Sheen argued psychoanalysis did not allow a person to live in the present, to use reason to apprehend the world around them. There was no objective reality.

Sheen told a joke to illustrate his point. Two psychoanalysts passed each other as they walked down the street. One said, "Good morning," and the other thought, "I wonder what he meant by that…" (Connelly, 1957). Sheen saw a slippery slope where all words and actions were fundamentally meaningless (without God) until given meaning by a human authority.

The third and final difference is that the normal person represses the "excesses" of the lower instincts in order to express reason and will and his "potential for divine grace" (Connelly, 1957). The repression for the abnormal person is the repression of reason and will to express the instincts. Sheen argued, "There is never a repression without an expression." By repressing instincts, reason can operate. By repressing reason, instincts dominate life.

As Sheen raised his voice, he declared, "Our nature is not that of a goat or a pig. Our nature is rational. We're human beings. Governed not by the subconscious mind…governed by a reason and by a will" (Connelly, 1957). Yet if human nature is rational, from where do the instincts and passions come? How do they figure into human nature as defined by being made in the image of God?

Yet Sheen acknowledged conflict is inevitable in life. "The greatest cross in this world," argued Sheen, "is to be without a cross" (Connelly, 1957). For Sheen, that personal, intrapsychic conflict is representative of the wider cosmic conflict between good and evil, obedience to God and sin against God. Sheen evidently made use of terminology and concepts such as repression, sublimation, and the subconscious, but attributed their dynamic to unique medical pathology, not the psychopathology of everyday life. Neurotic conflict, an experience for a select few, was for Sheen only aided by a life of faith engaged in the sacramental economy governed by the Church.

Not all Leuven graduates and faculty were as vehement in their criticism of psychoanalysis as Bishop Sheen. Born in Zwevegem, Belgium, Father Joseph Nuttin (1906–1988) was ordained in 1938, completed his PhD at the Katholieke Universiteit Leuven in 1941, and became a full professor in 1946. He spent his entire career in Leuven. While he is most known for his work with causality perception and cognitive reinforcement, he was well read in psychoanalysis and wrote multiple texts on the subject.

Around the same time Bishop Sheen was televising his program, Father Nuttin published *Psychanalyse et conception spiritualiste de l'homme* (Psychoanalysis and the Spiritualist Conception of Man, 1955). Another text, *Psychoanalysis and Personality: A Dynamic Theory of Normal Personality* (1962), was translated into English and went through multiple editions.

Nuttin distinguished the scientific theory of psychoanalysis from the *weltanschauung* or worldview that Freud and some of his followers had expanded the theory into. Nuttin identified the *weltanschauung* as the strongest barrier to religious acceptance of psychoanalysis. The clinical theory could be accepted in a narrow sense, a small component of what it means to be human. Integration for Nuttin meant pruning psychoanalytic theory to its fundamental clinical and scientific claims and picking and choosing the pieces seen as most valuable.

> The time has come to consider psychoanalysis as an ordinary scientific system, and this with a sufficient critical sense. This position means that we must not neglect the important objective data that psychoanalysis provides us for the reason that, often, the framework of interpretation exceeds the limits of a justified explanation, or because its total conception of man does not agree with our way of seeing.
>
> (Nuttin, 1955, p. 53)

Nuttin recognized the growth and development of psychoanalytic theory within Freud's work and that of his students. This theory was not a single system to criticize, as it was for Sheen, but a dynamic exploration of the mind which branched out in differing directions, some helpful, some not. "Integrating and situating psychoanalysis in the whole of science and psychological methods is the first objective we have assigned ourselves," wrote Nuttin (1955, p. 5). Thus, there was a fundamental difference between Father Nuttin and Bishop Sheen as they approached psychoanalysis. Sheen viewed psychoanalysis as a dangerous competitor to Catholicism and sought to show how psychoanalysis was a poor substitute for the real thing. Nuttin took a more complex view. He saw value in parts of the system but felt no need to adopt it as a whole.

Nuttin explained Freud's tripartite psychic system of the id, ego, and superego. Nuttin (1955, p. 57) took issue with his understanding of Freud's idea that the ego, developmentally, is constructed after the id, and is derived in part from the id, with the function of restraint for the drives of the id. Nuttin appreciated developments after Freud, especially by Franz Alexander and Anna Freud, which privileged the ego above the id. "Currently, we can say that it is the ego, and no longer the id, which is at the center of psychoanalytic theory" (Nuttin, 1955, p. 57).

Nuttin appreciated the shift away from the focus on unconscious drives, especially the libido theory, of psychoanalysis, and the promotion of ego psychology. He was as critical of the notion of the superego as he was the id. He appealed to Kant's cognitive perspective to dismiss the Freudian idea that moral judgment was connected to an emotional experience (for example, arousal or disgust). These arguments echoed the speeches of Pius XII in his encouragement for psychologists to focus on conscious self-control.

This criticism of the three agencies of psychic life is ineluctably tied to the notion of the unconscious overall. Nuttin (1955, p. 136) recognized how the theory of unconscious psychological conflict "profoundly changed the traditional and spiritualist image of man." The mechanisms Freud identified in this conflict interrogated the line between normal and pathological. "Thus, depth psychology collapsed from their pedestal the image of the royal man that the Renaissance had built, as well as the idol of the rational man of Age of Enlightenment" (Nuttin, 1955, p. 136).

Nuttin's most important observation, however, and the one that distinguished him from almost all other early Catholic readers of Freud, is that he saw no contradiction between unconscious conflict and human freedom endowed by God.

> It is not so much the conscious or unconscious source of the need as the felt need itself and its influence on behavior that are of interest here. In free behavior, in fact, the person takes a position with respect to the various elements of "value," or motives, insofar as they are currently experienced in the given situation; that is, insofar as these values constitute the object of an experience.
>
> (Nuttin, 1955, p. 149)

Nuttin argued that the decision about whether to engage in an action is determined consciously by the person in the moment. They may not have awareness of an unconscious motive, but they experience something consciously in their thoughts or their bodies. The person decides based on that experience.

> The "attractive power" or value of each motive is a function of the aspirations and impulses as they are experienced at the moment. The deeper source of these aspirations and impulses does not directly enter into the assessment of the motives or the subject's position with respect to them. In other words, it is to the extent that they are currently "felt" that the "motives" constitute forces that influence free behavior. Ignorance regarding their source changes nothing in the givens of the situation.
>
> (Nuttin, 1955, p. 149)

The individual may have an unconscious desire to have sex with another person, and this motive obviously does not enter the conscious decision-making of the individual. Yet their consciousness is not empty in the moment, there are emotions and thoughts and bodily sensations which the person uses to decide.

> The character of freedom or determinism of the act will now depend on the way in which the dynamic factors experienced within the subject

> trigger the activity. The act will not be free when the "motives" or drives cause the reaction to emerge as a link in the materially determined course of a natural process. It will, on the contrary, be free conduct when the subject finds himself confronted with the motives as elements of value that he recognizes intellectually, without being completely "absorbed" by their action on him.
>
> (Nuttin, 1955, p. 149)

Nuttin argued that a free act is one in which the person can recognize the varied motives influencing his decision. Nuttin seemed to suggest a balance between an intellectual understanding and an emotional acceptance. An act is not free when the person does not intentionally reflect and thoughtfully decide whether to act, instead allowing their impulses to run roughshod and dictate their actions.

Importantly, Nuttin (1955, p. 149) recognized that such a process is an ethical act. When the individual makes a free act, "he consciously consents to the motives that he himself values according to the concrete scale of values that constitutes his own personality." The free act is determined within the larger context of the person's value system. The free act is not random but fits a larger pattern.

> What we have just said shows that acts emanating from an unconscious dynamic source do not pose any special problem in terms of freedom. As with all other acts, whether they are free or necessary depends on whether the dynamism that drives one to perform the act has been worked out and implemented at the spiritual level of psychic activity.
>
> (Nuttin, 1955, p. 149)

Nuttin (1955, p. 162) seemed to define a free act by the extent to which one has justified their decision to themselves after due consideration of the potential motives affecting that decision. An act is free and moral when the individual assumes responsibility for the act and is the "author" of the decision.

Nuttin was remarkable for his connection and distinction between the aims of psychotherapy and morality, between the interventions of psychotherapists and moralists (in his profession, priests). Nuttin (1955, p. 166) argued psychotherapists help the (neurotic) patient "relax" their often-rigid views of themselves and others, and that, on the other hand, priests want to "fight against impulsive tendencies" and pursue the "conquest of an ideal personality." In so doing, "the moralist therefore considers the relaxation of the psychic effort constitutes a great danger."

However, Nuttin (1955, p. 166) warned, "the pursuit of an ideal is the most constructive but also the most destructive force that animates the human psyche." Nuttin did not seem to realize that when he wrote of a constructive and destructive ideal, he described the range of the superego, an agency he rejected earlier. Nuttin did not claim a solution to this tension between the need to restrict some impulses and relax others. He believed a balance could be achieved between the moralist and the psychotherapist.

Jacques Lacan and his "Discourse to Catholics"

Canon Henri Van Camp, professor of philosophy, theology, psychology, and psychoanalysis at the Facultés Universitaires Saint-Louis (a campus in Brussels historically tied to Leuven) invited the French psychoanalyst Jacques Lacan (1901–1981) to give two lectures to students and faculty during the spring of 1960. Lacan's lectures occurred within an ongoing series on philosophy and religion during that academic year.

Van Camp's invitation came roughly six weeks before the start of Lacan's annual seminar at St. Anne Hospital in November 1959, which would be published later as *The Ethics of Psychoanalysis.* Therefore, Lacan proposed his lectures in Brussels to be an extension of this topic, and the event shared the same title of the seminar. These two lectures took place between March 9–10, 1960.

At the start of his seventh seminar at St. Anne Hospital, Lacan (1986, pp. 2–3) outlined why psychoanalysis is "submerged" in the domain of ethics, both regarding its implied "ideal of conduct" and its corresponding "transgressions" of such conduct. Lacan therefore staked a significant claim somewhat aligned with Father Nuttin and against that of Maryse Choisy: psychoanalysis is a discipline of ethics.

Lacan (1986, p. 3) argued the primary contribution of psychoanalysis to the field of ethics is attention to the "omnipotence of a sense of guilt." Unlike Pius XII, who argued for absolution of guilt, Lacan did not seek to "soften, blunt, or attenuate the sense of guilt." Instead, Lacan wanted to explicate the connection between guilt and desire. Psychoanalysis "restored to favor...the productive function of desire." The papal attempt to limit the exploration and elaboration of desire, in effect, functioned as the censor which energizes desire.

Lacan continued this argument in Brussels. He did not want to proselytize or defend psychoanalysis. Where Pius XII sought to dismiss or limit psychoanalysis based on Catholic moral teaching, Lacan sought to show how psychoanalysis expanded or advanced the concept of morality in dialogue with Christian teaching. In January 1959, Pope John XIII announced his desire for a Second Vatican Council focused on "updating" the Church in dialogue with the world (covered in the next chapter). Lacan (2013, p. 11) argued that psychoanalysis's contribution to this dialogue is its conceptualization of human desire, "a new object for ethical reflection."

What connects desire to guilt? Lacan referred to Freud's (1964) myth of the primordial horde in *Totem and Taboo* which underpinned his concept of the Oedipal Complex. "Guilt finds its roots at the unconscious level, where it is linked to a fundamental crime for which no one can individually answer, nor has to" (Lacan, 2013, p. 30). This fundamental crime is the murder of the father of the horde by his sons, for the purpose of gaining access to the mother. The living father prohibited the sons from doing so and this prohibition was ineffective.

Desire for the mother led to the murder of the father, and the guilt about this murder led to the creation of the phobic object. This phobic object – the dead father – created distance between the horde and the object of their desire (Freud, 1964, pp. 132–146). Desire, what the Church considered to be the most offensive concept in psychoanalysis, was for Lacan the key to a sustainable ethics. Lacan's use of desire is almost always meant to be understood as *unconscious* desire (Evans, 1996, p. 37). Pius XII advocated a *conscious* effort at progressive growth through the repression of destabilizing forces. In this regard, Pius XII idealized the role of the ego in moral development.

Lacan (2013, p. 9) considered the focus on the ego, as well as "consciousness," "evolution," and "behavior," to all be reductive attempts at understanding and controlling human existence. Lacan was adamantly opposed to ego psychology, so appreciated by Father Nuttin and popular in the United States at the time. Lacan (2013, p. 9) stated:

> Nothing in the concrete life of a single individual allows us to ground the idea that such a finality directs his life and could lead him – through the pathways of progressive self-consciousness undergirded by natural development – to harmony with himself as well as to approval from the world on which his happiness depends.

If Nuttin, Sheen, and other Catholic theologians rejected psychoanalysis due to unconscious determinism, Lacan rejected the idea that consciousness alone has a natural determination towards a particular good. The symptoms which analysands bring to the consulting room are testaments to the failures of the pathways of progressive self-consciousness. Lacan spoke to the audience in Brussels about this unhappiness. Freud, and psychoanalysis, had something to offer to this problem in the conceptualization of the unconscious. Conscious, good intentions to live by moral standards or abide by religious protocols are not enough to satisfy the guilt which arises from the struggle to do so.

Lacan used – as he did during his seminar – St. Paul's *Letter to the Romans* to bolster this argument. Paul wrote, "If it had not been for the law, I would not have known sin" (Romans 7:7). In other words, the law, the moral commandments, make possible the desire to sin. The commandments in some sense activate or make one aware of the lost object. In this way, the ten commandments function as an external pleasure principle. "It is to the extent that the function of the pleasure principle is to make man always search for what he has to find again, but which he will never attain…" (Lacan, 1986, p. 68). Sin offers a concrete substitute object for the individual to "find," and even when found, does not satisfy. Hence the dissatisfaction.

While Lacan ended his reference to Romans at verse 11, verses 18–19 are relevant as well. Paul wrote, "I can will what is right, but I cannot do it. For I do not do the good I want, but the evil I do not want is what I do." This conflict is precisely what Lacan (2013, p. 23) articulated to his audience in Brussels when he stated desire is "diametrically opposed to intention." Again, Lacan contradicted the valorization of free will by Pius XII and Bishop Sheen. Conscious intention is problematized by unconscious desire. Guilt is structural to human experience, not something which can be absolved.

The impossibility for consciousness to lead to harmony, Lacan argued, is because the desired object – *das Ding*, the Thing – resides in the register of the Real, that aspect of experience which cannot be symbolized or articulated. The Church, according to Lacan, has no tool to address the Real other than to saturate it with meaning so that it can be ignored. The Church's Holy – living – Father continued to prohibit desire, and these prohibitions remained as ineffective in restraining human behavior as the primal father. The Real persists.

Lacan (2013, pp. 11–12) argued these experiences rooted in the unconscious need to be "translated" or "deciphered." To the extent possible, unconscious desire must be consciously, verbally articulated by the individual. The Church is ill-equipped for supporting such work, hence why Lacan titled this first lecture "Regarding Morality, Freud Has What It Takes."

Lacan focused in his second lecture on the biblical commandment "you shall love your neighbor as yourself" (Lev. 19:18). This commandment was one of two commandments (the other being to love God) which Jesus considered the greatest commandments (Mark 12:30).

Pius XII also addressed this commandment in his 1953 address. He insisted on

> a defense, an esteem, a love and a service of one's personal self, which is not only justified but demanded by psychology and morality. It is a natural evidence and a lesson of the Christian faith…Christ, then, proposes as the rule of love of neighbor charity towards oneself, not the contrary.
> (Pius XII, 1953, para. 12)

Pius XII implied psychoanalytic theory involved the opposite – a degradation of the self rather than charity.

This single commandment is therefore two commandments: love your neighbor but, to do so, first love yourself. Lacan went further than Freud's consideration of this self-love as being a representation of narcissism. Lacan questioned the self that is to be loved. The self is not merely comprised of the body, "but an image that misleads me by showing me my body in its *Gestalt*, its form" (Lacan, 2013, p. 33). People, insofar as they love themselves, love an image of themselves. This cohesive image is a cover for the otherwise fragmentary human experience.

Hence why Lacan (2013, p. 34) argued, "I love myself insofar as I essentially misrecognize myself – I merely love an other." The identifications which layer this image are grounded in the "structure" which is "already there before the subject begins to speak" (Lacan, 2013, p. 41).

Altruism – the love of one's neighbor – is thus the "transferring" of self-love to the other. How can an individual and their neighbors be led to harmony when the images they hold of themselves cover over psychic disharmony? As Lacan (2013, p. 40) argued:

> Man knows at the origin that he subsists in a relationship of ignorance, which means that man's psyche involves a first division by which everything with which he resonates...leaves out and skirts the Thing to which everything he experiences...is destined.

The fundamental split at the heart of subjectivity and the ignorance of this split prevents such harmony from developing. The Thing "marks the place where he suffers" the reality that "something is irremediably awry in human sexuality" (Lacan, 2013, pp. 42–43).

Lacan (2013, p. 47) identified a "gaping place from which the nothing questions us about our sex and our existence." People cannot love themselves or others based on a delusional harmony. Instead, this suffering "is the place where we have to love the neighbor as ourselves, because in him this place is the same" (Lacan, 2013, p. 47). Rather than deny or cover over the suffering necessarily entailed by repeated search for the Thing, our acceptance of it, through speech, offers a path forward.

This acceptance – this way of loving oneself and one's neighbors – is complicated by hate, the correlative to love. Lacan (2013, pp. 50–51) recognized people try to "compromise" with the Thing: through representations in art, through obedience to religious doctrine, and through scientific advancement.

These compromise formations attempt to reduce the tension the Thing exacerbates in the unconscious. Alternatively, Lacan argued psychoanalysis facilitates sublimation, a concept he elaborated in his seminar leading up to and following his lectures in Brussels. Rather than reinforce the faltering repression through compromise, sublimation allows the analysand to cultivate these tensions, to treat them as a starting point for more generative work. Sublimation will be discussed in chapter four.

The Triumph of Religion

This discourse between Catholicism and psychoanalysis, vacillating between hostile, ambivalent, and conditionally supportive, was well represented in Paolo Sorrentino's television drama, *The Young Pope* (2016). In one scene, the fictional Pius XIII (portrayed by Jude Law) argued with Cardinal Spencer (portrayed by James Cromwell) about how Church doctrine on abortion shifted over time as it incorporated developments in scientific knowledge.

PIUS XIII: "Science is the gift of God and God taught us that ovulation is spontaneous."

CARDINAL SPENCER: "Ask a woman about that: back when it was still believed that there were two kinds of insemination, male insemination involving sperm, female insemination involving eggs, it was considered a sin not to give a woman pleasure. But then, when it was discovered that ovulation was spontaneous, the cost was several billion female orgasms."

PIUS XIII: "But it made the psychoanalysts rich."

CARDINAL SPENCER: "The one profession that involves no work and a great deal of money that we let slip through our fingers."

(Sorrentino & Conterello, 2016)

Lacan spoke to this contention between science and religion in his *Discourse to Catholics*. Lacan stated:

> There is a certain flippancy in the way science disposes of a field regarding which it is not clear how it can so easily lighten its load. Similarly, faith has, a bit too often for my taste, been letting science resolve problems when questions translate into suffering that is a bit too hard to handle.
>
> (2013, p. 19)

On the one hand, the discoveries of science can make Church doctrine obsolete without any positive effect for religious people. On the other hand, the Church has often allowed scientific research to address suffering that threatens the Church's stability.

This arrangement between religion and science sometimes fails. It is in the gap of these failures that psychoanalysis is relevant. Lacan facilitated a press conference in 1974 which has since been titled "The Triumph of Religion." Lacan (2013, p. 65) argued, "Psychoanalysis did not arise at just any old historical moment. It arose correlative to a major step, to a certain step forward made by scientific discourse…psychoanalysis is a symptom." Scientific discoveries which revealed truth in opposition to the Church were responsible for the compromise formation of the symptom of psychoanalysis.

Lacan (2013, p. 8) argued, "Psychoanalysis is concerned especially with what doesn't work…the real is the difference between what works and what doesn't work. What works is the world. The real is what doesn't work." As he articulated in his *Discourse to Catholics*, people are "caught between the rational and the real," between knowledge and that which is not knowable (2013, p. 8).

To take the example provided by *The Young Pope*, through the determination that female pleasure is not required for fertilization, and the subsequent loss in orgasms, the Real intruded into the world and made things not work. The persistence of the Real is what problematizes the Church's meaning. The Real is a problem which often emerges due to science. Therefore, psychoanalysis is a symptom of the Real.

Lacan made a broad prediction. He argued that while psychoanalysis has managed a foothold of sorts, religion will eventually "excrete" enough meaning to cover over the Real. "If science works at it, the real will expand and religion will thereby have still more reasons to soothe people's hearts" (Lacan, 2013, p. 64). Science will continue to pursue truth without thinking through the consequences of its discoveries. And "somebody is going to have to give meaning to all the distressing things science is going to introduce" (Lacan, 2013, p. 64).

That somebody is the Church, which can "give meaning to absolutely anything whatsoever" (Lacan, 2013, pp. 64–65). Rather than distinguish the moralist from the psychotherapist in terms of restriction and freedom, Lacan reframed the conversation as one between the construction of meaning and its interrogation.

Any problem, any symptom, can be given meaning. "By drowning the symptom in meaning, in religious meaning naturally, people will manage to repress it" (Lacan, 2013, p. 67). The Church's view, and Lacan seemed to share it, is that the Church began with a place of prominence, its meaning was primary and without question. Eventually, science emerged and discovered all sorts of problems with Church doctrine. Some of these problems the Church handled through its excretion of meaning, some it could not handle. In this gap, the Real had an impact and psychoanalysis emerged. Lacan argued the Church would eventually excrete enough meaning to repress the symptom, cover the Real, and make psychoanalysis irrelevant. As Lacan (2013, p. 72) argued, "Religion is designed for that, to cure men – in other words, so that they do not perceive what is not going well."

About the beginning of this dynamic, Lacan referred to the Gospel of John. "The drama only begins when the Word is involved, when it is incarnated…It is when the Word is incarnated that things really start going badly. Man is no longer at all happy…Man is ravaged by the Word" (Lacan, 2013, p. 74). Ravaged is an interesting word, as Pius XII used it to describe the dangers of making the unconscious sexual desires, conscious. Lacan argued man is "ravaged" not by the "the impetuous flow of human thought and will" but by the Word the Church claims as source of salvation. In the end, rather than attempt to cover it over, Lacan (2013, p. 77) argued "we must be able to get used to the real."

Pope Francis and the Real

The papacy of Francis challenged these predictions. Joseph Bergoglio began his theological studies in Argentina in 1967. When Paul VI spoke warmly of psychoanalysis in 1973, Bergoglio took his final vows as a Jesuit. Around the time Lacan was in Rome delivering his press conference in 1974, the Dirty War began in Argentina when Bergoglio served as provincial superior.

The Dirty War was a period of nine years in which the government's military junta (supported by the United States as part of Operation Condor) led a reign of terror against anyone suspected of leftist political leanings which resulted in around "19,000 shot down in the streets, 30,000 'disappeared' and presumed dead (among them approximately 500 children), untold thousands imprisoned, and perhaps as many as two million Argentinians who went into exile" (Scavo, 2014, p. xi).

Multiple priests were among those killed, arrested, and disappeared. Bergoglio struggled to know how best to respond. Bergoglio reported he worked behind the scenes to protect those in need (Morello, 2015, p. 80). Indirect assistance was not enough for those who wanted public leadership. When his friend Alicia Oliveira, a former Attorney General of Argentina, urged him to speak out at the time, "he said he couldn't. That it wasn't an easy thing to do" (Miroff, 2013). Bergoglio could not speak.

About halfway through the war, Bergoglio sought the help of a Jewish, female psychoanalyst. As Pope Francis, he later told an interviewer, "For six months, I went to her once a week to clear up certain things" (Francis & Wolton, 2018, p. 273). He went to a psychoanalyst and spoke. The war ended in 1983, and by that time Bergoglio reportedly helped to save at least 100 people (Scavo, 2014).

Decades later, in that same interview, Pope Francis offered a generally positive view of psychoanalysis. When his interviewer, the French sociologist Dominique Wolton, referred to psychoanalysts as "pretentious," Francis disagreed, and stated, "I've also known some who were very human, very open to humanism and to dialogue with other sciences as well…The ones I've known helped me a lot in my life when I needed to consult someone" (Francis & Wolton, 2018, p. 273). Francis appeared to value psychoanalysts who engaged in dialogue and, like the analyst he once saw in Argentina, "stayed in her lane" (Francis & Wolton, 2018, p. 273).

The incarnation, and its loss, bring a confrontation with what is not working in the world. In other words, voicing lack and desire brings a confrontation with the Real. Like psychoanalysis, Francis wanted the Church to be concerned "especially with what doesn't work," the people and areas to which Jesus drew attention during his ministry. Jesus was a symptom of the Real. Such a perspective directs the work of the Church to where the symptoms lead: on the margins where the repressed places and people reside. The Church needs to speak about what is not working in the world and, simultaneously, listen to the voices of those who have not been heard.

Francis (2013, para. 191) wrote in his first Apostolic Exhortation, *Evangelii Gaudium*:

> In all places and circumstances, Christians, with the help of their pastors, are called to hear the cry of the poor…Seeing their poverty, hearing their

> cries and knowing their sufferings, we are scandalized because we know that there is enough food for everyone, and that hunger is the result of a poor distribution of goods and income.

Christians are called to listen.

Francis wanted the Church and its members to be scandalized by the suffering caused by what is not working in the world: the inequality driven by capitalism (Davies, 2013), the industrial damage to the climate and environment (Francis, 2015), the growing number of refugees (Glatz, 2023), and the destructive consequences of war (Pullella, 2022). As Francis (2014, p. 118) wrote:

> To this world it doesn't matter if many families have nothing to eat, do not have the dignity of bringing bread home; it doesn't matter that many people are forced to flee slavery, hunger, and flee in search of freedom. With how much pain, how often don't we see that they meet with death… the spirit of the world causes these things.

Therefore, alongside Lacan's stated need for people to "get used to the Real," Francis emphasized the need for mercy. From the beginning of his papacy, Francis appeared to shift the locus of Catholic morality away from judgment of immoral behaviors and practices of others towards a responsibility for Christians. Francis enacted this mercy himself.

During his first Holy Week as pope, rather than continue the tradition of washing the feet of Cardinals at the Vatican on Holy Thursday, Francis traveled to a juvenile detention center to wash the feet of inmates, including two women, one of whom was Muslim (Peralta, 2013). Where many of the predecessors of Francis practiced Catholic morality through its enforcement of canon law, which distanced them from the people under judgment, Francis wanted a Church which moved closer to those struggling with the conditions of their lives and world.

References

Baines, M. (2025). De Peccato Originali (On Original Sin 1679). *Intellectual History Review*, 35(2): 359–361. doi:10.1080/17496977.2024.2347074

Brown, S.J. (1927). Cardinal Mercier of Malines, 1851–1926. *The Irish Monthly*, 55 (651): 460–467.

Connelly, M. (Writer and Producer). (1956). Psychoanalytic couch (Season 5) [TV series episode]. In W. McDonnell, Sr. (Executive Producer), *Life is Worth Living*. Media City Teleproductions.

Connelly, M. (Writer and Producer). (1957). How to psychoanalyze yourself (Season 5) [TV series episode]. In W. McDonnell, Sr. (Executive Producer), *Life is Worth Living*. Media City Teleproductions.

Davies, L. (2013, December 15). Pope says he is not a Marxist, but defends criticism of capitalism. *The Guardian*. https://www.theguardian.com/world/2013/dec/15/pope-francis-defends-criticism-of-capitalism-not-marxist.

Dennis, P. (2020). Bishop Fulton J. Sheen: America's public critic of psychoanalysis, 1947–1957. *Journal of the History of the Behavioral Sciences*, 56(1): 36–51.

Evans, D. (1996). *An introductory dictionary of Lacanian psychoanalysis*. Routledge.

Francis (2013). *Evangelii gaudium* [Apostolic Exhortation]. Vatican. https://www.vatican.va/content/francesco/en/apost_exhortations/documents/papa-francesco_esortazione-ap_20131124_evangelii-gaudium.html.

Francis (2014). *The church of mercy: A vision for the church*. Loyola Press.

Francis (2015). *Laudato si'* [Encyclical]. Vatican. https://www.vatican.va/content/francesco/en/encyclicals/documents/papa-francesco_20150524_enciclica-laudato-si.html.

Francis. (2024). *Meeting with university teachers in the Katholieke Universiteit Leuven*. [Speech]. Vatican. https://press.vatican.va/content/salastampa/en/bollettino/pubblico/2024/09/27/240927c.html.

Francis & Wolton, D. (2018). *A future of faith: The path of change in politics and society*. St. Martin's Essentials.

Freud, S. (1953). The interpretation of dreams. In J. Strachey (Ed. & Trans.), *The standard edition of the complete psychological works of Sigmund Freud*, Vol. 4 (pp. 1–338). Hogarth Press. (Original work published 1900)

Freud, S. (1964). Totem and taboo: Some points of agreement between the mental lives of savages and neurotics. In J. Strachey (Ed. & Trans.), *The standard edition of the complete psychological works of Sigmund Freud*, Vol. 13 (vii–162). (Original work published 1913)

Glatz, C. (2023, March 21). Welcoming migrants, refugees is first step toward peace, pope says. *Catholic News Service*. https://www.usccb.org/news/2023/welcoming-migrants-refugees-first-step-toward-peace-pope-says.

Lacan, J. (1986). *The seminar of Jacques Lacan, Book VII: The ethics of psychoanalysis 1959–1960*. (J.A. Miller, Ed. & D. Porter, Trans.). Norton.

Lacan, J. (2013). *The triumph of religion: Preceded by discourse to Catholics*. (B. Fink, Trans.). Polity Press. (Original publication 2005)

Mercier, D. (1897). *Les origines de la psychologie contemporaine*. Institut Supérieur de Philosophie.

Miroff, N. (2013, March 13). Pope's role in dirty war under scrutiny. *The Washington Post*. https://www.washingtonpost.com/world/europe/popes-role-in-dirty-war-under-scrutiny/2013/03/15/53d6e3e6-8da3-11e2-b63f-f53fb9f2fcb4_story.html.

Misiak, H. & Staudt, V. (1954). *Catholics in psychology: A historical survey*. McGraw-Hill.

Morello, G. (2015). *The Catholic Church and Argentina's Dirty War*. Oxford University Press.

Nuttin, J. (1955). *Psychanalyse et conception spiritualiste de l'homme*. Publications Universitaires de Louvain.

Nuttin, J. (1962). *Psychoanalysis and personality: A dynamic theory of normal personality*. (G. Lamb, Trans.). Sheed & Ward. (Original work published 1953)

Peralta, E. (2013, March 28). In ritual, Pope Francis washes the feet of young inmates, women. *National Public Radio*. https://www.npr.org/sections/thetwo-way/2013/03/28/175601237/in-ritual-pope-francis-washes-the-feet-of-young-inmates-women#:~:text=During%20a%20Holy%20Thursday%20ritual,was%20a%20break.%20with%20tradition.

Pius XII (1953). *Speech by Pope Pius XII to participants in the international congress of psychotherapy and clinical psychology.* https://www.papalencyclicals.net/pius12/p12psyre.htm.

Pullella, P. (2022, February 25). Departing from protocol, pope goes to Russian embassy over Ukraine. *Reuters.* https://www.reuters.com/world/pope-went-russian-embassy-express-concern-over-war-moscow-envoy-2022-02-25/.

Scavo, N. (2014). *Bergoglio's list: How a young Francis defied a dictatorship and saved dozens of lives.* Saint Benedict Press.

Sheen, F. (1949). *Peace of soul.* McGraw-Hill.

Sheen, F. (1980). *Treasures in clay: The autobiography of Fulton J. Sheen.* Doubleday.

Smith, A.B. (1997). Prime-time Catholicism in 1950s America: Fulton J. Sheen and "life is worth living". *U.S. Catholic Historian*, 15(3): 57–74.

Sorrentino, P. (Writer & Director) & Conterello, U. (Writer). (2016, November 18). Season 1, Episode 9 [TV series episode]. In R. Amoroso (Executive Producer), *The Young Pope.* Wildside, Haut et Court TV, Mediapro.

Chapter 3

Psychoanalytic *Aggiornamento* and the Second Vatican Council

Pope Pius XII died in 1958 and with his death ended the "long 19th century," an era for the Catholic Church which started with the French Revolution in 1789. The phrase was coined by Soviet writer Ilya Ehrenburg to end with the outbreak of the First World War (Getz, 2018) but extended by O'Malley (2008) to include the death of Pius XII and the shift in the stance of the Church towards the world.

Pius XII wanted the Church to have persuasive counterarguments to the modernism, liberalism, and historicism movements which emerged from the Enlightenment and, in his mind, threatened the supremacy and truth of the Church. Psychoanalysis is best situated under the heading of modernism and, as previous chapters made clear, was something the Church thought needed to be opposed.

Then came the papacy of Pope John XXIII. When John XXIII first addressed the Second Vatican Council, two terms oriented the work of the participants: *aggiornamento* (bring up to date) and pastoral (a counterpart to doctrinal). Thus John XXIII (1962, para. 27) stated:

> The substance of the ancient doctrine of the deposit of faith is one thing, and the way in which it is presented is another. And it is the latter that must be taken into great consideration with patience if necessary, everything being measured in the forms and proportions of a magisterium which is predominantly pastoral in character.

Both of these terms are central to the collaboration possible between psychoanalysis and Catholicism. Psychoanalysis is a process of change, bringing up to date the psyche of the analysand. Where the neurotic analysand acts out a repetition of a forgotten past there is a calcification of meaning (Freud, 1964a). The analyst as pastor accompanies the patient in their suffering, responds to their demand for change, and does not dictate the outcome of that change.

In its institutional neurosis, the Church had become, for John XXIII, a storehouse for antiquities of doctrine, stuck in a repetition of doctrine that

DOI: 10.4324/9781003485346-4

had lost its efficacy. The Catholic theologian Hans Küng (1979, pp. 96–98) agreed with Freud's criticisms of religion when Freud observed the "defective forms of religion," "the churches' misuse of power," and the "traditional image of God." Küng, a significant participant in Vatican II, well understood the stakes at play.

> When religion is manifested in rigid fidelity to the letter, in a legalistic conscience, in obsessive, pedantic and petty repetition of certain prayers, formulas, and rituals, religious ideas come close to delusive fabrications, religious observances to substitute satisfaction resulting from obsessive cultic repetition.
>
> (Küng, 1979, p. 97)

Pope John XXIII wanted the Magisterium to be primarily pastoral, that is, not rigid, not legalistic, and not obsessive. He stated just prior to his election: "We are not here to guard a museum, but to cultivate a flourishing garden of life" (Barron, 2014, p. 170). A museum, full of dead people and inert objects, does not change. A garden is a site defined by change and growth, the expansion of life.

The argument here was not whether the Church should change. Without doubt, the Church has changed time and again (see Noonan, 2005, on the development of Catholic moral teaching). The concern of John XXIII was the Church's posture towards change. Was change something to be guarded against or welcomed into the life of the Church? John XXIII firmly planted himself in the latter camp.

This chapter therefore explores how psychoanalysis was discussed during Vatican II and argues *aggiornamento* and psychoanalysis go hand in hand in their shared pastoral ministry in solidarity with a suffering world. Events which preceded the Council and coincided with it help illustrate how the Church shifted from opposition to ambivalence in its ongoing engagement with psychoanalysis.

While the Council did not cite psychoanalysis in its final constitutions and decrees, the text most relevant to this discussion is *Gaudium et Spes* (Flannery, 1996). The lesson is that the Church cannot change on its own, set apart from the world, in an echo chamber. *Aggiornamento* requires an Other.

For the analysand, the Other is the analyst. For the Church, the Other is the world. Whereas the Council reaffirmed its recognition of "two orders of knowledge," faith and reason, psychoanalysis insists on a third: the unconscious. Each order only makes sense and is beneficial to the individual alongside the others.

Preceding the Council

One document issued during the preparatory period before the Council was the *Religiosorum Institutio: Instruction on the Careful Selection and Training of Candidates for The States of Perfection and Sacred Orders* (February 2, 1961).

This document outlined the requirements for selecting and training priests, monks, and nuns. It also addressed problems which commonly occurred in the process at that time. In doing so, it made use of psychoanalytic concepts.

For example, candidates who "defect" do so because they "unconsciously transfer" their "present state of mind and psychic crisis" to "their profession and ordination, being unaware of the inner change which has taken place within themselves" (John XXIII, 1961, para. 12). Without fanfare, the Church found utility in the concept of the unconscious and put it to its own uses.

Diagnostic language was also used to identify who should be excluded from selection. The document identified "those who give evidence of neuropsychosis and who are described by psychiatrists as neurotics or psychopaths, especially those who are scrupulous, abulic, hysterical, or who suffer from some form of mental disease (schizophrenia, paranoia, etc.)" (John XXIII, 1961, para. 31).

Those potentially in treatment with a psychoanalyst should not be selected for the clergy! The Church recognized the profound psychic conflict at play in neurosis and psychosis and wanted that conflict as far away from the cloth as possible. The unconscious, so far as it existed, was not acceptable in the clergy.

The Church instead wanted "youths who are physically and psychically normal or endowed with good bodily and mental health, who are noted for solid piety and the other virtues intimately connected with chastity, and who sincerely desire the religious and priestly life" (John XXIII, 1961, para. 2). Freud's work disputed any notion of psychic normality. The extent to which desire can be "sincere," i.e., consciously intended, is what Lacan discussed the year prior.

Some clergy leaders used psychoanalysis to address this question of sincerity or desire in the process of selecting members for the clergy. Father Gregoire Lemercier (1912–1987) was a priest born in Liege, Belgium, and entered monastic life in Leuven, Belgium, in 1932. After the Second World War, his Mexican peer Ignacio Romerovargas Yturbide convinced him to move to Mexico, and, with the permission of Pope Pius XII, he founded a Benedictine monastery (Fernández-Cobián, 2024). After the installment of Sergio Méndez Arceo (1907–1992) as Bishop of Cuernavaca, St. Mary of the Resurrection was founded near Cuernavaca, Mexico.

While Lemercier was already familiar with psychoanalysis and had recommended some of his monks to attend, he did not attend psychoanalysis until he experienced a frightening hallucination. His personal experience as an analysand led him to believe everyone in the monastery could benefit from the process. In what Gallo (2011, p. 219) called "the most eccentric episode in the Mexican reception of psychoanalysis," Lemercier initiated a requirement which used group psychoanalysis to encourage candidates or even established monks to discuss potential unconscious motivations for their desire for religious life.

However, Lemercier's interest in bringing analysis to the monks was not entirely selfless. After accepting nearly anyone who wanted to become novices, Lemercier "soon realized that the community had become filled with maladjusted and violent characters – drug addicts and active homosexuals, above all – who compromised the climate of prayer and intellectual work" (Fernández-Cobián, 2024, p. 7). His fantasy of an ideal monastery was awash in symptoms!

While Lemercier deeply appreciated psychoanalysis, and believed in its capacity to aid spiritual formation, he seemed to want to use it to cleanse his community of what he perceived to be sin. Homosexuality, something Freud considered "nothing to be ashamed of, no vice, no degradation" (Grotjahn, 1951, p. 331), was for Lemercier something to excise from the community. He doubted the calling of religious life for people with desires and behaviors he personally abhorred.

As Giniger (1967, p. 15) reported for *The New York Times*, "Since last September, Father Lemercier has been in Rome defending psychoanalysis as a method of solidifying the vocation of the monks and of barring of aspirants who have no real vocation and who might later show psychic disorders." Lemercier seemed to take an authoritative stance regarding the normative outcome for the group analysis as well as what made someone fit for monasticism. While apparently Freudian in his theory, he did not seem to consider the psychopathology of everyday religious life to be an existential to accept and work through but something to exclude.

During this experiment, approximately 40 candidates and monks, out of a total of 60, left the monastery ("Benedictine on trial," 1966, p. 15). When news of this experiment spread, the Vatican responded. A *Monitum* (warning) against the attendance at or practice of psychoanalysis by Church officials was issued in July 1961. It read, in part:

> Clerics and religious are forbidden to practice psychoanalysis…The opinion of those who consider that a prior psychoanalytical examination is definitely necessary before receiving Holy Orders must be disapproved. Likewise disapproved are the opinions of those who hold that the so-called psychoanalytical examination and relative investigations are necessary for candidates to the priesthood and for religious profession. This applies also if it is a matter of investigating the aptitude required for the priesthood or for religious profession. Likewise, the priests and men or women religious must not go to psychoanalysts except with the permission of the Ordinary and then only for grave reasons.
>
> ("Psychoanalysis off limits," 1961, p. 5)

To what extent the *Monitum* was an attack on the practice of psychoanalysis was debated. While some read the *Monitum* as a direct response to psychoanalysis, others argued, "The Holy Office has indicated no opposition to psychoanalysis; it is merely protecting its proper application" ("Clerics and psychoanalysis", 1961, p. 4). The question of proper application was not a mere excuse. After all, Lemercier initiated this practice with virtually no oversight/supervision, no formal training himself, and without initiation on the part of the monk patients.

After Bishop Arceo pleaded the case of psychoanalysis during Vatican II (see more details below), Lemercier traveled to Rome in September 1963 to attempt to force a confrontation with the authorities who challenged his work. The Holy Office declined to see him but reminded him of his duty to obey the *Monitum* (Fernández-Cobián, 2024, p. 10). Lemercier continued his experiment. He publicized the fight with the Vatican across newspapers and magazines and published his own pamphlets. Multiple investigations were facilitated with the awareness and approval of Pope Paul VI (Pope John XXIII having died in 1963). After a trial which he left partway through, Father Lemercier was convicted under canon law (O'Grady, 1967). The monastic community decided to close, and the members pursued various futures.

Lemercier requested and received dispensation for his vows at 55 years of age and married a woman. With those decisions, Lemercier completed his analysis and decided against commitment to religious life. While he attempted on a practical level to integrate spiritual discernment and psychoanalysis, his attitude towards those who interrogated his practice produced further divide.

Bishop Arceo, despite his steadfast support of Lemercier even through his wedding, lamented the tragedy of the community. "I am particularly concerned about the danger that psychoanalysis may have engendered an excessive confidence and become a new panacea, a substitute for religion" (Fernández-Cobián, 2024, p. 11). Surely this panacea was the fantasy of Lemercier who could not find in the end a way to integrate these dual vocations within himself.

Second Vatican Council

John XXIII shocked the Church and the world when he announced his plans for a Second Vatican Council. Before outlining the major changes inaugurated by this event, it is worth describing the theological landscape affirmed by the First Vatican Council. Vatican I, despite its name, was not the first council facilitated by the Pope. It was, in fact, the twentieth ecumenical council. Held between 1869–1870, this Council was initiated by Pope Pius IX in response to the rise of secular philosophy and morality through the Enlightenment priority of reason or rationalism.

Revelation, not reason, was the source of truth. Immanuel Kant's work had already been placed on the Index of Prohibited Books decades prior (Göbel, 2024) but the Enlightenment persisted, nonetheless. The Council declared human reason was a *component* of understanding truth revealed by the Pope through the power of the Holy Spirit. In response to modernity's diffusion of authority and knowledge, the Council insisted on the ultimate authority of the Magisterium and the supremacy of the Pope. This council defined the doctrine of papal infallibility.

The Council's answer to modernity was to revive (though with significant alternations) the philosophy of St. Thomas Aquinas. As the previous chapter described, this neo-Thomist project was initiated by Pope Leo XIII.

> The revival of neo-scholastic philosophy and especially of Thomism was perceived to be a suitable means for countering positivism, liberalism and emerging socialism. So, in order to offer an alternative to modern philosophical and political ideas, Leo XIII fell back on a medieval philosophical system.
>
> (Lamberts, 2021, p. 32)

The return to medieval philosophy was intended to find ammunition to fight modernity. Modernity was perceived as a threat to the Church. However, that strategy did not stop the Church's growing irrelevance to the secular world.

With the Curia willing and able to make changes to Church doctrine and practice and to produce responses to modern challenges, and with the infallibility of the pope affirmed during Vatican I, Bishop Butler (1974, p. 256) acknowledged the right to ask, "Why incur the trouble and expense of [another] ecumenical council?" His answer was that the Second Vatican Council intended something more than incremental policy decisions, that it sought more radical change.

> Such new solutions will have a radical quality and will entail a searching discrimination between what is, after all, of the immutable essence of the Church, and all in her contingent existence that, however venerable, is yet – at least in principle – expendable.
>
> (Butler, 1974, p. 258)

The tension between an immutable essence and what is expendable, or radically alterable, is a tension which exists in psychoanalysis as well. Is the symptom part of the essence of the individual's subjectivity or is the symptom something which can be radically altered? Is sexuality part of the immutable essence of human nature or is it something which can be expended? Is guilt something which can be absolutely absolved or something more ontological about being human? John XXIII's intention for the Council was to interrogate this tension in a fashion comparable to the process of psychoanalysis.

The framework for the process was oriented by three elements, "*aggiornamento*, *ressourcement*, and the development of doctrine" (Blanchard, 2022). Undergirding these terms was the pastoral posture. This chapter addresses *aggiornamento* while *ressourcement* is discussed in a later chapter. *Aggiornamento* is an Italian word which means update, or to bring something up to date. While Pope John XXIII initially used the term exclusively regarding canon law, the term eventually came to describe his desire for updating the Church at large: "*Aggiornamento* injected the problem of change into the council in an unavoidable way, but even without it, the problem of the relationship of past to present would most surely have arisen and been just as pervasive and troubling" (O'Malley, 2008, p. 9).

Change was a problem for a Church which expounded the infallibility of the Pope and the unchangeable, unquestionable, doctrine of the Magisterium. What change, then, did John want for the Church? The answer has been debated ever since the end of the Council. Mahieu (2012, p. xxix) summarized the position of Yves Congar, another key theologian during the Council, and stated:

> The Church must no longer look upon itself as a citadel, obsessed with the battle against enemy forces. It is called to enter into a true dialogue with the contemporary world, a dialogue that Congar did not envisage naively, as being without confrontations and arguments between the parties, but one in which both partners would enrich each other, the Church having its mission to proclaim the Gospel and to serve the world in accordance with this Gospel, the world leading the Church to question the Gospel anew, to purify itself continually and to develop its catholicity by welcoming new values. This Church…must show itself to be in solidarity with the world in its pilgrimage towards the Kingdom.

Thus, the Council was an incredible opportunity for the Church to partner, rather than parry, with psychoanalysis. Psychoanalysis, a process intended to produce change, can help to lead the Church to question the Gospel anew. To consider the goal of psychoanalysis to be an update in the psychic reality of the patient helps to clarify the update sought by Pope John XXIII. In other words, Catholicism after Vatican II and psychoanalysis after Lacan pursued a psychoanalytic *aggiornamento*. Bishop Butler (1974, p. 257) referred to the Council as "*aggiornamento* in depth." This chapter argues the present needs of the Church require *aggiornamento* with depth psychology.

While no official reference to psychoanalysis is made in the 16 official constitutions, decrees, and declarations (Flannery, 1996), the published *Acta Synodalia Sacrosancti Concilii Oecumenici Vaticani II* (Proceedings of the Synod of the Second Vatican Ecumenical Council) include several references, both minor and major, to Freud and psychoanalysis. The *Proceedings* include transcripts and written submissions of comments made by various bishops and other participants in the Council during the general congregations which discussed the drafting of the eventual 16 documents published by the Council.

In the first period of the Council, a schema was in development for a constitution on chastity, marriage, family, and virginity (*Schema Constitutionis Dogma Ticae De Castitate, Matrimonio, Familia, Virginitate*) (Concilio

Vaticano II, 1962). The schema was not a sign of a developing partnership. Unsigned, this document railed against the primacy of sexuality identified by psychoanalysis. The second chapter articulated a defense of chastity:

> They therefore seriously offend against the teaching of the Church, who assert that, even in a well-healthy man, almost everything, including the religious, the moral, and even the supernatural, must, as it were, be explained a priori from the sexual, with the added accusation that the shepherds of souls are to be considered unfit and incapable of their duty, if these and other modern they do not know the requirements.
>
> (Concilio Vaticano II, 1962, p. 724)

The document responded in part to unidentified writers who apparently accused the Church of being neglectful in its duties to parishioners if it did not educate its clergy on psychoanalytic insights into sexuality. But it primarily took issue with the psychoanalytic idea – which Lacan taught in Brussels – that sexuality is fundamentally disturbed in all people, not simply the psychoneurotic. In the footnotes, reference was made to the speeches by Pius XII detailed in chapter one.

However, the authors of this draft recognized the critical feedback Pius XII's speeches received in the footnotes of the schema. "The so-called pansexualism is not expressly touched upon here, since it is clear that today there are psychologists who deny that Freud himself really taught pansexualism" (Concilio Vaticano II, 1962, p. 730). The schema does not engage or even mention what Freud really taught and how that teaching could edify Catholic moral life. The authors detailed their attempt to strike a balance on the subject.

> It is clear that neither the Supreme Pontiff nor the present Constitution wants to condemn the knowledge and usefulness of these sciences, even among priests; However, it is a mistake to explain everything by sex in the pastoral care of souls, and to accuse the Catholic pastoral care as if in this matter the Church has failed in the essentials in regard to the direction of souls.
>
> (Concilio Vaticano II, 1962, p. 730)

In other words, the Catholic Church wanted to make use of constructive insights gained through psychoanalysis but disagreed with the idea that sexuality explained everything. Unfortunately, the authors of this schema did not elaborate on what they understood the "usefulness" of psychoanalysis to be. Instead, they argued psychoanalysis could not wholly condemn the Church for not accepting its every insight. The document was intended to condemn the "errors" and "exaggerations" of the sexual instinct as conceptualized by psychoanalysis. The schema's focus on errors and exaggerations missed the opportunity to acknowledge and explore the truths and applications of psychoanalytic theory.

Despite this attempt at threading the theoretical needle, further footnotes condemned specific theorists for their published work. Dr. Angélo Louis-Marie Hesnard (1886–1969) was a French psychoanalyst and one of the founding members of the Société Psychanalytique de Paris. Hesnard corresponded with Freud over the years, although their relationship was contentious due to Hesnard's disagreements with Freud (Roudinesco, 1990, p. 74). Hesnard also collaborated with Maryse Choisy, cited in chapter one, on her journal *Psyché*.

Hesnard was controversial within France, both for the perception of his work but also his defense of Lacan, and he eventually joined Lacan in the École Freudienne de Paris. Lacan (1986, p. 2) referenced Hesnard in his first session of *The Ethics of Psychoanalysis*. The Vatican document condemned Hesnard's best known book at the time, *Morality without Sin*, and noted the book was placed on the Vatican's *Index Librorum Prohibitorum*, its list of prohibited books (Concilio Vaticano II, 1962, p. 728). This note corresponded to the ongoing conflict with Hesnard in the wider church, particularly the criticism of Father Agostino Gemelli (referenced in chapter one) (Roudinesco, 1990, p. 200).

Alongside Hesnard, Father Marc Oraison, priest and psychoanalyst, was also condemned in this draft constitution (Concilio Vaticano II, 1962, p. 732), and likewise it noted his placement on the *Index Librorum Prohibitorum* for his 1951 book *Christian Life and the Problems of Sexuality*. In 1970, Oraison was attacked by a "mob" of "French traditionalists" outside the Church of Notre Dame de l'Assomption in Paris ("French traditionalists mob Oraison," 1970, p. 1). The repression of Hesnard and Oraison is addressed in the second section of this book.

The draft of this constitution was rejected by the Council (de Mattei, 2018, p. 3) and no reference is made to Pius XII's 1952 and 1953 addresses in any of the later approved constitutions, decrees, and declarations. John XXIII died in June 1963 and was succeeded by Paul VI. Psychoanalysis is not discussed again at the Council for another two years.

Brief references were made in October 1964. Bishop Gasbarri compared Freudianism to other secular, self-centered movements such as idealism, existentialism, and materialist communism (Concilio Vaticano II, 1964, p. 458). Bishop Kuharic spoke to "some confused opinions under the influence of Freudianism and hedonism of this time" which "call into question the divine teaching on the sanctity of conjugal life" (Concilio Vaticano II, 1964, p. 581). Bishop Osvaldo Salinas Fuenzalida included Freud alongside philosopher Jean-Paul Sartre, political theorist Karl Marx, and artist Pablo Picasso as a group of influential secular intellectuals which the Church needed its own group to oppose (Concilio Vaticano II, 1964, p. 663).

The last documented discussions of psychoanalysis during the Second Vatican Council were also its most positive. Bishop D'Souza referred to a colleague's admonition for the Church to avoid another trial like Galileo in its condemnations of other schools of thought.

> Last year, a certain honorable moderator exclaimed: one case of Galileo is enough. But in the meantime, we had, not to mention others, the case of Lammenais, the case of Darwin, the case of Marx, the case of Freud, and recently the case of Teilhard de Chardin. Of course, their works and the movements initiated by them were affected by some errors, but nevertheless they advocated the genuine values that our schema now recognizes. Why, then, were they to be condemned indiscriminately? Was not the word of scripture to be heard: "Prove all things, hold fast to what is good?"
>
> (Concilio Vaticano II, 1964, p. 478)

Bishop D'Souza argued that the admonition was too late, and the Church continued to repeat the same mistake time and again. By holding fast to what is good, he appealed to an appreciation of the complexity of psychoanalytic theory, accepting pieces which were in accord with Catholic teaching and rejecting the pieces which were opposed to doctrine.

Bishop Sergio Méndez Arceo strongly argued in favor of psychoanalysis to his colleagues. Bishop Arceo oversaw the diocese of Cuernavaca, where Father Lemercier had conducted his experiment in psychoanalysis. Arceo began with caution but quickly declared his stance:

> This science is not fully mature and still today involves risks that must be carefully considered; that is not why we can ignore the "psychoanalytic revolution," which is no less than revolution or technical change. The brilliant invention of Sigmund Freud is to be valued like the inventions of Copernicus or Darwin.
>
> (Concilio Vaticano II, 1965, pp. 626–627)

Bishop Arceo's references to Copernicus and Darwin, and later Galileo, warned the Council against making the same mistake with Freud as the Church made with these other scientists, whom they condemned for being against Church doctrine but later were forced to concede their truth. That which the Church had taught to be immutable, and severely punished those who disagreed with it, turned out to be adaptable to scientific progress.

Bishop Arceo continued that "the unconscious subject is in each one of us, in every human activity, whether religious, cultural, economic, or political, to manifest itself and, whether we like it or not, exercises its most effective influence," and in the end, there was "no field of pastoral activity where psycho-analysis should not be kept in mind, and in fact it is already being kept in mind by many" (Concilio Vaticano II, 1965, p. 627).

Bishop Arceo was specific when he described the "field of pastoral activity," the same connection made by Oskar Pfister and Sigmund Freud decades prior. Psychoanalysis is a pastoral activity which brings lived experience into dialogue with doctrine. Arceo argued that if the Council wanted, as part of its larger mission given to it by John XXIII, to speak with relevance and persuasion to the world at large, it must take psychoanalysis as a serious interlocutor.

Finally, Bishop Badré, in his written submission to the Council, appealed to the groundbreaking nature of psychoanalytic theory. Freud, he argued, "had the courage to defy the professional ethics of Viennese doctors by publishing the 'Dora case.' Without this audacity, medicine would not have the precious resources of psychoanalysis to treat mental disorders" (Concilio Vaticano II, 1965, p. 1013). The audacious nature of Freud's work was essential to its development. To be offended by his defiance is to misunderstand the nature of what makes scientific progress possible.

News reports at the time also indicated psychoanalysis was a significant topic of conversation among the bishops during the Council (Schneider, 2024). For example, Father Jerome Hayden, O.S.B. was a monk and psychiatrist asked by Cardinal Suenens to present to the Council in the fall of 1964 on his views on psychoanalysis and Catholicism (Hayden, 1967; Seitz, 2015). Father Hayden was the founder and director of the Marsalin Institute in Massachusetts, a psychiatric facility which sought to demonstrate the compatibility of psychoanalytic theory with Catholic doctrine. Father Hayden completed his theological studies at the University of Leuven.

His remarks were not included in the formal documents from the Council but were instead relayed in Catholic newspapers and his later reflections on the Council. Father Hayden is reported to have said:

> If human behavior is not seen, appreciated and understood, and accordingly dealt with, in the light of present-day psychoanalytic discoveries, the *aggiornamento* set in course by Pope John and continued by Pope Paul will, in a very real sense, be a failure.
>
> (McCloskey, 1965, p. 5)

In this respect, Father Hayden aligned himself with Bishop Arceo in his insistence that the Church could either enter the dialogue with psychoanalysis or be left behind.

Father Hayden continued:

> If the Church refuses to perform this task, it will nevertheless be undertaken without her. We would then find ourselves in a contradictory situation in which the teachings of Christ would be appropriated and incorporated into a "new" moral science proposed outside the Church.
>
> (McCloskey, 1965, p. 5)

Father Hayden identified morality, ethics, as the central point of either collaboration or conflict between Catholicism and psychoanalysis. The Church could either play ball, or forfeit the match, but it could not win without engagement with psychoanalysis. The Council instead appeared to play to a draw. The Council concluded in December 1965 without any mention of, let alone a formal position on, psychoanalysis.

The silence continued for eight years until Paul VI (1973) spoke about psychoanalysis during a general audience. He stated its importance in society had become clear.

> We have an esteem of this now famous current of anthropological studies, although we do not always find them consistent with each other, nor always validated by satisfactory and beneficial experiences, nor supplemented by that science of hearts, which we draw at the school of Catholic spirituality.
>
> (Paul VI, 1973, para. 5)

His words were neither a stirring endorsement nor a condemnation of psychoanalysis.

Gaudium et Spes

While no document issued by the Council addressed psychoanalysis, the *Constitution on the Church in the Modern World* referred to psychology. This Constitution was unique in its length, depth, and scope. It was also one of the only documents to have no prior template in the schemas created in preparation for the Council. *Gaudium et Spes* emerged from the dialogue at the Council, which is why Reverend McGrath (1966, p. 397) concluded "this Constitution is that of the Council itself." It represented the culmination of the Council and, for those who did not see the work of the Council as finished in 1963, the Constitution was a roadmap to encounter the world moving forward. Psychoanalysis was part of the world the Church needed to encounter if its *aggiornamento* was to be fulfilled.

The Constitution tied effective evangelization to an astute understanding of the world.

> In every age, the church carries the responsibility of reading the signs of the times and of interpreting them in the light of the Gospel, if it is to carry out its task...We must be aware of and understand the aspirations, the yearnings, and the often dramatic features of the world in which we live.
>
> (Flannery, 1996, p. 165)

The Church must listen to and learn about the secular world, about the people living in it, if it expects to have an active role. "Reading the signs of the times" is an ambiguous phrase and continues to be the subject of debate. What is meant by "reading" and what is meant by "signs" is certainly open. At the very least, if the Church is reading, the Church is not talking. If the Church is attentive to signs, it means the meaning of those phenomena is not immediately clear. The Constitution therefore insists the Church must maintain an overall posture of humility towards the world.

The Constitution recognized the Church must listen to the advances in understanding the human psyche made possible by psychology. "At no time have people had such a keen sense of freedom, only to be faced by new forms of social and psychological slavery" (Flannery, 1996, p. 166). Freedom versus slavery is an important Christian dichotomy, from the subjugation of the Israelites in Egypt to the slavery of sin poignantly described by St. Paul.

This specific tension is explored at length in chapter five. Without explicit reference to psychoanalysis, the Council here acknowledged the profound experience of psychic conflict and the projection and expression of this conflict in the social sphere. As Canon Moeller (1966, p. 415) described in his commentary on the Constitution:

> The text of the Constitution insists that the disorders existing in the world are not only due to "technical defects," to accidental errors in organization, but are rooted more deeply in an inclination to evil which splits man within himself. This is what sin is, the fundamental disorder that human remedies can never completely heal.

This passage almost reads like Bishop Sheen's argument articulated in the previous chapter. However, the difference is important. Sheen took a posture of already knowing the reality about which psychology claimed to discover. He claimed psychic conflict was simply a secular way of understanding sin and removing the spiritual aspect from it. He learned nothing new from it and saw only a secular discipline taking authority away from the Church.

However, the existence of the ontological split within humanity is inevitably to be represented in, but not equated to, the psyche of each individual. The unconscious conflict within the psyche of an individual does not map perfectly onto the conflict between good and evil. The phenomenon of scrupulosity is enough evidence in this regard. The psychoanalytic notion of psychic conflict is one representation or manifestation (alongside others, such as war) of this ontological conflict.

Therefore, despite the continued insistence on the unity of an individual, that is, between body and soul, the Council recognized of the conflict in the individual, and how disciplines other than theology and biblical hermeneutics, like psychology and sociology, have knowledge it needs to fully understand how the ontological conflict plays out in the world today, and how to effectively address it.

The Constitution continued. "Advances in biology, psychology, and the social sciences not only lead humanity to greater self-awareness, but provide it with the technical means of molding the lives of whole societies as well" (Flannery, 1996, p. 166). Psychology has produced not only knowledge of the mind, but knowledge about how to produce change. This knowledge and corresponding mechanisms of change are developed apart from the Church. The Church aims to change people, to help people become more like Christ. The Council wanted the Church to make use of psychology in its mission of discipleship.

In doing so, there was a recognition of the connection between the pastoral and the psychotherapeutic methods.

> In pastoral care, sufficient use should be made, not only of theological principles, but also of the findings of the secular sciences, especially of psychology and sociology: in this way the faithful will be brought to a purer and more mature life of faith.
>
> (Flannery, 1996, p. 239)

Though "sufficient use" is ambiguous, the effectiveness is not: The Council argued that through the application of psychology, Christians would develop purity and maturity. Far from danger to the faithful, psychology was seen as a necessary aid on the path to holiness.

Unfortunately, despite this collaborative framework, the Council provided only one clear example of how it wanted to make use of psychology: reinforcement of doctrine on marriage and the family, particularly conjugal love.

> Experts in other sciences, particularly biology, medicine, social science and psychology, can help secure the welfare of marriage, the family and people's peace of mind if by pooling their findings they try to clarify thoroughly the different conditions favoring the proper regulation of births.
>
> (Flannery, 1996, p. 227)

Here is where the difference between psychoanalysis and psychology comes into focus for the Church. Psychoanalysis is a method of interrogation of conscious beliefs and statements. Change occurs through the unconscious becoming conscious. Psychology, particularly behaviorism, is a method of reinforcement. Change occurs through the association between a targeted behavior and a reward or punishment. Psychoanalysis says that people – including the leaders of the Church – have less conscious control of their thoughts and actions than they think they do. Behaviorism says the opposite: people are more in control of themselves than they think. Governed for centuries by a system of laws which required strict obedience, the Church has always been more comfortable with the theory of behaviorism versus psychoanalysis. The implications of this preference and difference are discussed at length in section two of this book.

Psychoanalysis has nothing to contribute to how conception and birth should be regulated, nor does it proscribe an ideal family structure. It does, however, have something to contribute to understanding the *desire* to regulate these phenomena. Psychoanalysis does have something to say about the *ideals* the Church wants its members and clergy to strive for in certain issues but find themselves time and again falling short of achieving for themselves: monogamy, procreation, abortion, sexual orientation, dignity, etc.

Conclusion

The shift away from explicitly discussing psychoanalysis and the challenges it raised to the Church towards a general acceptance of psychology insofar as it reinforced existing doctrine was a disappointing step away from the potential of *aggiornamento*. Given the debates detailed above, no doubt it would have been difficult if not impossible to achieve consensus on any declaration about psychoanalysis. This tension was obviously not new. As Canon Moeller (1966, p. 421) put it:

> The relations between the Church and culture have never been idyllic. One has only to remember the case of Galileo. However, even these difficulties can and should promote a more profound diffusion of the Church; they raise new questions that require new research on the part of theologians. (Think, for example, of the problems raised by psychoanalysis).

Whereas much ink has been spilled on the tension between religion and science, the Council recognized a more pervasive and consequential tension between Church and Culture. A capital C is used here to emphasize the centrality of culture to the subjectivity of the human person. "Culture belongs to the essence of the human person. It is not something superfluous that one can do without; it leads to true and full humanity" (Moeller, 1966, p. 419). Culture is not one constructed aspect of materialism subsumed under the authority of the Church but is stitched into the psyche of each person.

The Council took a broad approach when it defined culture. "The word 'culture' in the general sense refers to all those things which go to the refining and developing of humanity's diverse mental and physical endowments" (Flannery, 1996, p. 229). While broad, by using words like "refining" and "developing," the Council's definition paints culture with a positive hue. Such a framework adheres to the theory of cognitive/evolutionary psychology which maligns primitive mental functioning and idealizes civilized rationality.

Again, the Church's fundamental values (distinct from revealed truth), are used and reinforced without question. "Culture, since it flows from humanity's rational and social nature, has continual need of proper freedom of development and a legitimate possibility of autonomy according to its own principles" (Flannery, 1996, p. 235). That the Council's understanding of culture excluded irrationality and passion betrayed the degree to which they were committed to a Scholastic philosophy of the higher order of humanity. The Second Vatican Council reinforced the First Vatican Council's determination of "two orders of knowledge" (Flannery, 1996, p. 235), faith and reason.

Sigmund Freud (1964b, p. 219) once detailed his theory of two orders of knowledge, or as he put it, two principles of mental functioning. In the beginning of psychic development was primary process governed by the *pleasure-unpleasure principle*. This principle governs the pursuit of pleasure and the avoidance of unpleasure. The mechanism of repression enables the mind to split off whatever is unpleasurable and create a psychic reality full of pleasure. External reality is rejected. Fantasies and dreams are examples of the pleasure principle.

As time passes, the individual is unable to sustain complete and consistent pleasure within psychic reality, the individual gains more agency, and the mind engages with external reality and attempts to change it. Hence, the *reality principle* is the second principle of mental functioning (Freud, 1964b, p. 219). The question undergirding both principles is how the individual decides to manage their psychological unpleasure or pain. Although more complicated that this simple picture, the pleasure principle is mostly unconscious while the reality principle is mostly conscious.

Importantly, Freud did not make a judgment about the reality principle being more important or ethically better than the pleasure principle. The goal of psychoanalysis was not and is not to eliminate the pleasure principle. After all, the desire and search for pleasure, or as philosophers often term it, "the good," is an important and necessary drive in human nature.

Freud was clear that these principles coexist in the psychologically mature individual. Repression is an imperfect mechanism both because it is always only partially successful and the superego is not always judging based on an objective moral compass. Therefore, one cannot trust that whatever desire is repressed is in accordance with Catholic moral teaching. There is a need to continually interrogate the conscious mind and its justifications for repressing desire. The Council debates did not address or resolve how the Church needs to update itself with this fundamental aspect of Freud's work.

The two orders of knowledge outlined by the Councils inspired by St. Thomas Aquinas already encompass the reality principle with its consciousness, reason, and appeal to external reality. Psychoanalytic *aggiornamento*, however, insists on a third order of knowledge: the unconscious, where the pleasure principle operates. This order of knowledge is not within the scope of the Church or based in the supernatural, as is faith, and is not quantifiable and deducible, like reason. The unconscious is defined in part by being in opposition to the other orders. The unconscious is not based on external or lived reality. The unconscious calls reason and faith into question.

Each of these orders is independent and yet holds the others accountable. Without faith, reason and the unconscious are too self-centered, that is, the mind is too preoccupied with itself. Faith provides humility through the recognition of God's authority, knowledge, and grace. Without reason, faith and the unconscious have no contact with reality. Cut adrift from lived experience, and no practice of logic, the risk of psychotic religiosity emerges.

Without the unconscious, faith and reason take themselves too literally, too concretely, too much at face value. There is an arrogance that comes with the dismissal of the unconscious, a devotion to an idol of self-knowledge which perpetuates repetition compulsion.

Aggiornamento is therefore an ongoing task of the Church as it encounters the world of psychoanalysis. Many issues continue to confront the Church 60 years after the Second Vatican Council which psychoanalysis is in a unique position to help address: sexuality and gender (sexual abuse, chastity, sexual orientation, pregnancy and abortion), the formation of priests and the dramatic decrease in the number of active clergy, authority and hierarchy within the Church and its relation to the world, and more. The final two sections of this book are an attempt to put this psychoanalytic *aggiornamento* into practice.

References

Barron, R. (2014). *Catholicism: A journey to the heart of faith*. Random House.

Benedictine on trial for psychoanalysis. (1966, December 16). *The Catholic Transcript*. Retrieved from the Catholic News Archive.

Blanchard, S. (2022). The reform was real: Continuity and change at Vatican II. *Commonweal Magazine*. https://www.commonwealmagazine.org/reform-was-real.

Butler, B. (1974). *Searchings*. Geoffrey Chapman Publishers.

Clerics and psychoanalysis. (1961, August 3). *The Pittsburgh Catholic*. Retrieved from The Catholic News Archive.

Concilio Vaticano II. (1962). *Acta synodalia*, Vol. 1. Vatican.

Concilio Vaticano II. (1964). *Acta synodalia*, Vol. 3. Vatican.

Concilio Vaticano II. (1965). *Acta synodalia*, Vol. 4. Vatican.

de Mattei, R. (2018). Humanae vitae and veritatis splendor, rooted in the perennial Magisterium of the Catholic Church. Paper given at the JAHLF Conference, Rome, May 21.

Fernández-Cobián, E. (2024). Psychoanalysis, religion and architecture. Fray Gabriel Chávez de la Mora and the monastery of Santa María de la Resurrección. *Hispania Sacra*, 76(154): 1–20.

Flannery, A. (1996). *Vatican Council II: The basic sixteen documents*. Costello Publishing Company.

For priests, religious: Psychoanalysis off limits. (1961, July 21). *The Monitor*. Retrieved from The Catholic News Archive.

French traditionalists mob Oraison, Laurentin. (1970, February 4). *National Catholic Reporter*, 6(14): 1.

Freud, S. (1964a). Remembering, repeating and working-through. In J. Strachey (Ed. & Trans.), *The standard edition of the complete psychological works of Sigmund Freud*, Vol. 12 (pp. 145–156). Hogarth Press. (Original work published 1914)

Freud, S. (1964b). Formulations on the two principles of mental functioning. In J. Strachey (Ed. & Trans.), *The standard edition of the complete psychological works of Sigmund Freud*, Vol. 12 (pp. 213–226). Hogarth Press. (Original work published 1911)

Gallo, R. (2011). Freud's Mexican readers. *Psychoanalysis & History*, 13(2): 207–225.

Getz, T. (2018). *The long nineteenth century, 1750–1914: Crucible of modernity (the making of the modern world)*. Bloomsbury Academic.
Giniger, H. (1967, September 6). A monastery in Mexico closed in dispute over psychoanalysis. *The New York Times.* https://www.nytimes.com/1967/09/06/archives/a-monastery-in-mexico-closed-in-dispute-over-psychoanalysis.html.
Göbel, C. (2024). A dark chapter: Revisiting the Church's censorship of Kant. *Commonweal Magazine.* https://www.commonwealmagazine.org/dark-chapter.
Grotjahn, M. (1951). Historical notes: A letter from Freud. *International Journal of Psychoanalysis*, 32: 331.
Hayden, J. (1967). *Religion and psychiatry: A historical perspective.* Marsalin Institute.
John XXIII (1961). *Religiosorum institutio: Instruction on the careful selection and training of candidates for the states of perfection and sacred orders.* Sacred Congregation For Religious. https://adoremus.org/1961/02/religiosorum-institutio/.
John XXIII (1962). *Solemn opening of the Second Vatican Council.* [Speech]. Vatican. https://www.vatican.va/content/john-xxiii/es/speeches/1962/documents/hf_j-xxiii_spe_19621011_opening-council.html.
Küng, H. (1979). *Freud and the problem of God.* (E. Quinn, Trans.). Yale University Press.
Lacan, J. (1986). *The seminar of Jacques Lacan, Book VII: The ethics of psychoanalysis 1959–1960.* (J.A. Miller, Ed. & D. Porter, Trans.). Norton.
Lamberts, E. (2021). Religious, political, and social settings of the revival of Thomism, 1870–1960. In W. Decock, B. Raymaekers, & P. Heyrman (Eds.), *Neo-Thomism in action: Law and society reshaped by neo-scholastic philosophy 1880–1960* (pp. 29–40). Leuven University Press.
Mahieu, E. (2012). Introduction. In Y. Congar, *My journal of the Council.* (M. Ronayne & M. Boulding, Trans.). Liturgical Press.
McCloskey, P. (1965, January 9). Acceptance of psychiatry by church held vital. *Catholic News Service, Newsfeeds.*
McGrath, M. (1966). The Constitution on the church in the modern world. In J. Miller (Ed.), *Vatican II: An interfaith appraisal* (pp. 397–412). University of Notre Dame Press.
Moeller, C. (1966). Man, the church and society. In J. Miller (Ed.), *Vatican II: An interfaith appraisal* (pp. 413–421). University of Notre Dame Press.
Noonan, J. (2005). *A church that can and cannot change: The development of Catholic moral teaching*. University of Notre Dame Press.
O'Grady, D. (1967, May 31). Vatican curbs monk psychoanalyst. *National Catholic Reporter.*
O'Malley, J. (2008). *What happened at Vatican II.* The Belknap Press of Harvard University Press.
Paul VI (1973). *General audience.* Vatican. https://www.vatican.va/content/paul-vi/it/audiences/1973/documents/hf_p-vi_aud_19731107.html.
Roudinesco, E. (1990). *Jacques Lacan & co.: A history of psychoanalysis in France, 1925–1985.* Chicago University Press.
Schneider, A. (2024). "Making the holy obscene": A thematic analysis of Freudian psychoanalysis in the Catholic press. *Integratus*, 2(1): 13–36.

Part 2

Theory and Theology

Chapter 4

Repressive Censorship versus Merciful Sublimation

One cannot speak of the unconscious without speaking about repression. Repression is one mechanism which splits the conscious and unconscious mind. "The essence of repression," Freud (1957b, p. 147) wrote, "lies simply in turning something away, and keeping it at a distance, from the conscious." Freud used the analogy of "ordering an undesirable guest out of my drawing room" and having a "permanent guard over the door" to prevent further access (Freud, 1957b, p. 153). This permanent guard is the censor who rejects a potential guest based on judgment. Freud concluded this censor is the psychic agency of the superego.

Censorship is a longstanding practice of the Catholic Church, as represented by its Index of Prohibited Books. The Index was the result of investigations by the Holy Office into authors and texts considered dangerous to the souls of Catholics (Vose, 2022). Through placement on the Index, Catholics were prohibited from purchasing, owning, or reading these texts. The Index was an expression of the Church's repression driven by its institutional superego.

Sexuality was a core subject of censorship. This chapter explores the work of two psychoanalytic authors who were placed on the Index – Dr. Angelo Hesnard and Father Marc Oraison – at a time when sexual abuse perpetrated by the clergy was ongoing. Church censorship of sexuality did not prevent sexual harm. Repression, as Freud taught, is only ever partially successful. What is repressed always returns.

Pope Francis reoriented Catholic morality around mercy. His infamous reflection, "Who am I to judge?" was representative of his pastoral practice (Winfield, 2013). Censorship and repression are opposed to mercy because censorship requires the harsh judgment of the superego and forces desire to operate unconsciously. As Pope Francis (2016, p. 52) taught: "The Church does not exist to condemn people but to bring about an encounter with the visceral love of God's mercy." Instead, the psychoanalytic notion of sublimation is a strategy to accept and direct desire towards what is constructive. Blind obedience to the law needs to give way to merciful sublimation.

DOI: 10.4324/9781003485346-6

Psychoanalytic Repression

Freud provided his most comprehensive explanation of the mechanism in his paper "Repression" (1957b). Freud detailed how repression is the result of conflict. While the instinct seeks satisfaction, there are "other claims and intentions" which would produce dissatisfaction (Freud, 1957b, p. 147). In this conflict, "the motive force of unpleasure shall have acquired more strength than the pleasure obtained from satisfaction" (Freud, 1957b, p. 147). Repression is the result of the fear of unpleasure being stronger than the desire for satisfaction. The mind has no choice but to address this conflict as "the ego cannot escape from itself" (Freud, 1957b, p. 146).

Freud distinguished between three phases of repression. First, prior to the development of the superego, in early infantile life, Freud (1957b, p. 148) presumed "primal repression" to exist. Primal repression is a basic experience of the psychical representation of the instinct being "denied" entry to consciousness (Freud, 1957b, p. 148).

Repression proper is the second phase. Any images, words, or memories which are associated with basic instincts are potentially subject to repression. Freud (1957b, p. 148) described the repulsion of the law driving the image to be repressed but also how what is already repressed exerts a pull on those potential associations into the unconscious. One may think of a black hole, pulling into its orbit objects which are being simultaneously driven towards it.

However, unlike the objects pulled into a black hole, the phenomena which are repressed continue to exist. Repression "interferes" only with the conscious system of the mind (Freud, 1957b, p. 149). Now located within the unconscious system, the thoughts and images are free to develop and express themselves into "extreme forms" which, when confronted with them in consciousness, the individual does not recognize them at all (Freud, 1957b, p. 149). Freud wrote, "This deceptive strength of an instinct is the result of uninhibited development in phantasy and of the damming-up consequent on frustrated satisfaction" (1957b p. 149).

Left to the unconscious, the instincts and their corresponding representations, held back from satisfaction, intensify in a way that is less likely when they are conscious. While Freud (1961) argued repression of the instincts such as uninhibited aggression and sexual desire is the basis for a peaceful, rational civilization, civilization comes at a significant psychological cost. Repression of the libido contributes to the formation of symptoms and repression of aggression contributes to the experience of guilt (Freud, 1961, p. 139).

Religion, for Freud, was a significant partner of repression and aimed to help distance the instincts from consciousness. When Pius XII (1953) taught "moral demands" dam "human thought and will" so that they do not "overflow" and "cause ravages," he advocated for the mechanism of repression. Yet Pius XII did not address the cost of this damming up of the instincts. He did not accept, as Freud (1957b, p. 151) taught, that "repression demands a persistent expenditure of force." The repressive dam is not a one-time construction which permanently restrains the instincts but a dynamic process which requires consistent maintenance.

Symptoms are not the product of repression per se but are "indications of the return of the repressed" (Freud, 1957b, p. 154). As Laplanche and Pontalis (1973, p. 398) put it, "repressed material not only escapes destruction, but it also has a permanent tendency to re-emerge in consciousness. It does so by more or less devious routes, and through the intermediary of secondary formation." The return of the repressed is therefore the third phase of repression.

Repression therefore shapes human behavior through distancing the instincts from consciousness according to the dictates of the superego. There is an ideal ego, an image of the kind of person an individual wants to become, which helps to frame what is repressed. There is no destruction of the id, of desire. Freud understood internal psychic conflict as a resolution of external Oedipal rivalry, which allowed for the development of civilization. Freud argued it is out of the internal tension that the sense of guilt arises.

Catholic Censorship

Publications by members of the clergy were required by Canon Law to be reviewed for congruence with Catholic doctrines. First, the clergy's local bishop designates a *Censor Librorum* (censor of books) to determine whether the text contained any content at odds with Catholic doctrine. If the text passes examination, it is deemed *nihil obstat*, or nothing hinders, the publication of the text. If the author was under the authority of a religious order such as a monastery, their major superior must review the text and conclude *imprimi potest*, it can be printed, moving it closer towards publication. Finally, the author's bishop provided the final approval, the *imprimatur*, let it be printed (Vose, 2022, p. 108).

These phrases or designations were then printed on the inside of the book, typically on the copyright page, and list the people who provided each of the designations. Such designations provided Catholic readers with the assurance that what they were reading was validated by the Church and allowed the texts to be used in Catholic education. Readers can continue to see these designations in books to this day.

Historically, while this process went through the local diocese of the author, the Supreme Sacred Congregation of the Holy Office (hereafter Holy Office) in Vatican City investigated texts alleged to be in violation of Canon Law. If it was deemed contrary to Church teaching, the text was recommended to be placed on the *Index Librorum Prohibitorum* or the Index of Prohibited Books. The Pope, in his role as the highest-ranking official in the Holy Office, made the final determination.

The Index was formalized in 1559, when the Holy Office was known as the Supreme Sacred Congregation of the Roman and Universal Inquisition, and continued until 1966 under Pope Paul VI, an astonishing 400 years of deep recognition, analysis, and censorship with literature across that time (Barbierato, 2022). The Index of Prohibited Books was one Index within the larger Indices which included laws and procedures for broader doctrinal questions and decisions of the Church which the Holy Office was designed to adjudicate and enforce.

One of the best illustrations of the danger of such censorship is the novel *The Name of the Rose* by Umberto Eco (2023). In the fourteenth century, a Benedictine abbey in Northern Italy was the host of a doctrinal conflict between the Vatican and the Franciscans. The Franciscans, true to their name, were living an extremely ascetic life of poverty to protest what they saw as the corrupt wealth and power of the Vatican.

William of Baskerville, a Franciscan friar, came to witness the debate with his apprentice Adso of Melk. They quickly become detectives when a monk is found dead, then another, then another. William and Adso discovered the murders were committed by a monk, Jorge, who wanted to keep secret the existence of a book in the abbey's restricted library: the lost second volume of Aristotle's *Poetics*, which taught the virtues of comedy and laughter.

Jorge covered the pages of the book in poison, killing those who touched it, to make literal his perception of its spiritual danger. In the end, he began to chew and swallow the pages of *Poetics* to prevent its dissemination. He set fire to the library and himself. Death and chaos, not life and order, was the result of his actions. William concluded:

> Fear prophets, Adso, and those prepared to die for the truth, for as a rule they make many others die with them, often before them, at times instead of them. Jorge did a diabolical thing because he loved his truth so lewdly that he dared anything in order to destroy falsehood.
>
> (Eco, 2023, p. 516)

What William saw in Jorge's actions was a perverse devotion to the law or, simply, legalism. Jorge believed he sought the common good of the community by censoring a poisonous text from being distributed and corrupting their minds. He never considered whether they could learn something from the text, whether there was anything in the text which would align with, reveal, or deepen Christian faith. He also ignored the particularities of the lives of his brother monks. He isolated himself in a tower, in dialogue only with his conscious thoughts.

Censorship of Angelo Hesnard

The Catholic Church engaged in significant censorship of psychoanalytic texts in the 1950s. Two authors of such texts are the focus of this chapter: the psychiatrist and psychoanalyst Dr. Angelo Louis Marie Hesnard (1886–1969) and the medical doctor and priest Reverend Dr. Marc Oraison (1914–1979). With Freud having died in 1939, both Hesnard and Oraison are important figures in psychoanalysis as they bridged its first and second generations.

Two books by Hesnard caught the attention of the Catholic Church. *l'Univers morbide de la faute* (The Morbid Universe of Guilt, 1949) and *Morale sans péché* (Morality without Sin, 1954) were censored by the Supreme Sacred Congregation of the Holy Office with the final approval of Pope Pius XII.

Hesnard elaborated in *Morbide* his conceptualization of psychopathology as a fundamentally moral problem. Hesnard understood that what afflicts the mind, so-called mental illness, is not a biological or chemical dysfunction but is rooted in moral conflict.

Hesnard (1949, p. 22) referred to this moral conflict as a "drama which unfolds before a phantom tribunal, in an imaginary courtroom, with an endlessly renewed, merciless indictment and a pleading without conclusions." Hesnard (1949, p. 291) wanted to remove all moralism from the study of psychopathology to reach a "foundation of a [secular] science of ethical behavior." Importantly, Hesnard (1949, p. 291) understood endogenous guilt to be, not a subjective affective phenomenon, but "as a structure, embedded in the very foundations of human behavior."

Hesnard interpreted the morbid guilt in the severe symptomatology of his mentally ill patients as belonging to all people. "Guilty behavior, in its elementary, obscure, and secret form, is an integral part of all human conduct" (Hesnard, 1949, p. 292). Despite the doctrine of original sin, the Church was invested in maintaining the medical distinction between mental wellness and illness because it reinforced the spiritual distinction of purity and depravity in the human person.

Hesnard (1949, p. 294) argued that what is considered authentic ethical behavior is often the result of forced renunciation of personal enjoyment due to the threat of vindictive punishment. Every interaction with another person, the Other, is driven by the desire to not be accused of guilt. Ethical behavior stems, then, from the historical experiences of prohibition and punishment (threatened or given) as well as the prophylactic effort to maintain innocence before the Other.

Hesnard understood people's actions were often motivated by the avoidance of guilt, of not wanting to suffer the aftermath of sin, and thereby sidestep punishment, rather than the desire to do good. The structural element of guilt predisposes the individual to act towards the prevention of fault and further guilt (Hesnard, 1949, p. 301). In essence, the forced obedience to a moral law exacerbates repetition compulsion. Behavior is thus unconsciously driven by an unreal sense of guilt which bypasses the reality principle of the ego.

This dynamic is the morbid universe of guilt Hesnard identified in moral law. This is why Hesnard (1949, pp. 300–301) concluded, "the only fruitful ethical attitude" is "doing better, drawing inspiration from the Guilt not to punish but to prevent its recurrence." The prevention of recurrence is the resolution of repetition compulsion.

The Holy Office commissioned a report authored by Father Philippe de la Trinité (born Jean Rambaud) to determine whether *l'Univers morbide de la faute* should be placed on the Index. Philippe (1954, p. 3) introduced his report with a balanced perspective, before ultimately determining that it should placed on the Index. "Despite the interest it presents from a psychological point of view (there is a non-moral pathological guilt), it contains enough obvious doctrinal errors…to have to be put on the Index."

What were these obvious doctrinal errors? Philippe, rather than provide commentary on the text, quoted about 14 passages of the book which he apparently thought would speak for themselves in terms of their heresy.

Philippe (1954, p. 4) quoted Hesnard: "Humanity wastes its time stubbornly trying to justify itself or accuse instead of acting, remedying, perfecting, creating. Guilt, Accusation, Sanction should be merely incidental occasions for examples, useful only for dealing with the base instinct of social vengeance." Hesnard gave common examples of people who, without prompting, make statements like "It's not my fault" or "He's to blame." Hesnard interpreted these experiences as representative of his thesis that there is an underlying strategy in avoiding or denying guilt.

In Philippe's role within the Holy Office, indeed in this very report on Hesnard, Philippe investigated an *accusation*, determined *guilt* of doctrinal error, and sought the *sanction* of censorship in the placement of the text on the Index. Hesnard understood this strategy unnecessarily reinforced that morbid universe of guilt. Censorship is therefore a core feature of the morbid universe of guilt.

Hesnard instead argued for acts of "remedying, perfecting, creating" in response to guilt. To take his book and the Holy Office as an example, Philippe could have engaged Hesnard in conversation and provided constructive criticism to the author. Hesnard could have had an opportunity to respond in further writing. The psychological value Philippe saw in the text could have been encouraged and matched by a clearer communication of his concerns regarding the theological impact.

The last passage worth reviewing here concerns sexuality, in particular, masturbation in adolescence. Philippe quoted a long passage in which Hesnard claimed masturbation is "most often more effect than cause" of the morbid universe of guilt (1954, p. 5). What he meant by "more effect than cause" was that the desire for sexual intercourse which many adolescents begin to experience prompts significant guilt and that guilt is often avoided through masturbation.

Hesnard argued masturbation violates natural law when it acts out "resistance to the attraction and then to the exercise of the normal sexual act" (Philippe, 1954, p. 5; Hesnard, 1949, p. 378). Hence, masturbation, or any sexual act, can aid the strategy to avoid guilt. Hesnard claimed that the nonmasturbator could also be in violation of the natural law because the refusal to masturbate may also be an attempt to avoid guilt.

This distinction allowed for a moral practice of masturbation. Church doctrine did not and does not allow for any masturbation, any sexual act outside of adult marriage. Hesnard's conception of morbid guilt and the avenues the mind takes to avoid it problematized the Church's black and white moral code. Rather than engage this critique with the aim of updating moral theology and edification of its readers, the Church chose to censor the text and prohibit its dissemination and availability among Catholic institutions.

Hesnard's sequel book, *Morality without Sin*, was "reported to the Holy Office as a proclamation of the failure of universal morals, including the Christian one" (Philippe, 1955, p. 2). Hesnard advocated a moral system not oriented around sin. The philosopher Paul Ricoeur, in his critical review of both texts, helpfully outlined Hesnard's definition of sin. "By sin, he doesn't mean the theological dimension of all guilt, that is to say the 'before God' and even the 'against God' of guilt" but rather addresses the "inauthentic manner of experiencing culpability" (Ricoeur, 1955, p. 342).

Hesnard wanted moral judgment to rest on acts, behaviors, and not internal dispositions or thoughts. Philippe (1955, p. 6), in this report, quoted a representative passage:

> The morality of the future, concrete because demystified, could be a morality without demon or taboo, without malignity of fate or superstition of destiny. A joyful and fertile morality coinciding with the authentic spirituality that Christianity conceived without yet being able to realize it: the action committed, and not dreamed.

Because the morbid morality of the superego was inevitably unreal in its construction and distorted in its judgments, Hesnard did not see a way for the psyche to house or utilize an authentic moral compass. This was a strange conclusion for a psychoanalyst to argue, because treatment theoretically aims at uncovering the desires and judgments in the unconscious to enable greater conscious freedom for the individual. Instead, Hesnard (1949, p. 165) focused on evil and moral *action* rather than sentiment (Philippe, 1955, p. 7).

The mental or internal sinner, for Hesnard, "lives in anguish not because of what he does but because of what he imagines himself to be" (Ricoeur, 1955, p. 342). This phenomenon is what Hesnard termed the "myth-morality of sin" (Hesnard, 1949, p. 42). Pathological guilt is the consequence of an internalized ideal of identity which the superego harshly judges as never being accomplished. For Hesnard, action is the only way to resolve this guilt.

Though Philippe (1955, p. 17) recommended this text be placed on the Index, he also recommended against a wholesale rejection of psychoanalysis:

> If a condemnation were indeed made, it would be necessary to avoid, in any possible unofficial commentary, casting discredit on psychoanalysis as such, because I believe, quite the contrary, that we owe a very great debt of gratitude to the Catholic thinkers and psychologists who work to separate the wheat from the chaff, from the psychoanalytic point of view. With its profoundly human psychology, Thomism can easily assimilate the valid contributions of psychoanalysis.

This conclusion is rather shocking. Written during the papacy of Pius XII, it reflected a clear acceptance of psychoanalysis in an official but private Vatican document not seen in any public writing.

Around the same time, prior to its placement on the Index, Father Agostino Gemelli (1955) took up Hesnard's *Morality without Sin*. Gemelli agreed with Hesnard's premise that there are people who suffer from internal guilt disconnected from reality. However, Gemelli argued this guilt is based on ignorance of God's love rather than instantiated by Church law.

"The moral situation of many Christians presents certain structural traits that the revelation of liberation from sin, of liberation from the regime of the Law, and of forgiveness in Jesus Christ, does not seem to have touched" (Gemelli, 1955, p. 2). Gemelli argued "educators and confessors" would benefit from understanding this moral situation of many Christians who seek their teaching and direction.

Gemelli (1955, p. 5) encouraged Catholic leaders to "ensure the authenticity" of the "aspirations" of Catholics in their spiritual journeys, whether in discipleship, religious life, or the priesthood.

> We must not confuse absolute, rigid, unintelligent obedience with voluntary submission to a superior; the cult of suffering can, in certain subjects, be the beginning of a morbid introversion which causes us to confuse the objects of our egocentrism with the ends of charity.
>
> (Gemelli, 1955, p. 5)

Hesnard would likely have agreed with this overall sentiment. However, psychoanalytic theory questions the belief in an objective standard of authenticity free from unconscious influence. Such a belief reflects and reproduces the rigid system Gemelli claimed to reject. Hesnard engaged in a similar rigidity when he opposed the interior and exterior life, between intention and act.

While Gemelli's conclusions are welcome, he failed to see how the Church has historically demanded the absolute, rigid, unintelligent obedience Gemelli rightly rejected. The Church, led by humans, is partly responsible for Christians being ignorant of their liberation of the regime of the law. Its practice of censorship, while at this time was limited to virulent reproaches and bookstore shelves, was simply a more civilized version of its historical barbaric violence directed at those with whom it disagreed (e.g. the Inquisition).

What Hesnard failed to realize is that the system he sought to change was reflective of the approach of church officials in history and not inherent and immutable Christian truth. Hesnard likewise failed to see, as Gemelli and Philippe noted, the inseparable connection between thought and action. Moral action, external, is always based on desire, which is internal. Hesnard seemed to imagine a morality not only without sin, but without the unconscious. Such a system has never been, and cannot be, realized.

Finally, it is important to note how little Hesnard discussed sublimation in his texts. In *Morality without Sin*, there is only one passing reference in an endnote. *The Morbid Universe of Guilt* contains six references with the only substantial discussion being about the moral importance of art (1949, p. 490). Hesnard did not engage with sublimation as an important component of psychoanalytic ethics.

Censorship of Marc Oraison

Marc Oraison (1914–1979) was a French Catholic priest and medical doctor who applied psychoanalytic theory to his work in spiritual direction and psychotherapy. Oraison's work is engaged here based on his early work on morality and sexuality.

Oraison trained as a surgeon before he entered seminary at 29 years of age. He detailed this early history in his memoir, *Strange Voyage: The Autobiography of a Non-Conformist* (1970). His medical training was purely biological, and he took no interest in psychiatry at that time. It was not until seminary at the Institut Catholique de Paris that he was introduced to psychoanalysis.

Oraison was in his early thirties when he enrolled in a course on moral theology with Father Eugéne Tesson, S.J. Oraison recalled:

> We all [Tesson included] sensed vaguely that its basic orientation was awry. Without being able to explain exactly why, we knew that this legalistic and abstract formulation of the laws of right and wrong was as far removed from the realities of human life as it was from the revelation of the Gospels.
>
> (Oraison, 1970, p. 145)

Tesson recommended Hesnard's work on sexology to the entire class.

Oraison's thesis was requested for publication even before he was finished. It became *Christian Life and Problems of Sexuality* (1951). Following its defense, the thesis earned him *prorsus cum singulari laude*, the "highest possible award" (Oraison, 1970, p. 156). Father Albert Plé, psychologist and priest, provided the *nihil obstat* for the book. Father Tesson wrote its preface.

To his surprise, Oraison was confronted by the Vatican while in Rome at a congress on psychoanalysis and theology. "On Thursday of Easter Week, I received a summons to appear before the Holy Office on Saturday, at eleven o'clock in the morning. The Holy Office's secret police had reported my presence in the City" (Oraison, 1970, p. 160). Legalism was afoot. In the 1950s, the doctrinal department had its own police force it used to track and detain clergymen it deemed a threat.

Two Cardinals were present when Oraison arrived: Cardinal Pizzardo, then the second-ranking member of the Holy Office (under the Pope), and Cardinal Ottaviani, his assistant.

> Pizzardo opened the conversation, and certain phrases have remained with me. The general idea was that my book was pernicious and aimed at subverting tradition, and it was dangerous to morals. In a good sexual education, the Cardinal said, the most important thing was fear of hell – supplemented by a solid diet of starches and pastas. This was especially true in the case of future priests. Here are Cardinal Pizzardo's words, verbatim: "For purity in the seminaries, we need fear, spaghetti, and beans."
>
> (Oraison, 1970, p. 161)

Fear, protein, and carbs were the only elements necessary for sexual education. Knowledge of the unconscious was superfluous. The Church wanted to instill fear of hell, not desire for heaven, in those confronted by sexuality in the modern era. This fear left no room for mercy.

The Holy Office requested Father Philippe and Reverend Sebastiano Tromp to read the text and provide their input. Father J. Geraud also provided extensive commentary on the text. The Holy Office received multiple letters which alleged Oraison's text was "seriously harmful to souls, especially those dedicated to the Lord in the priesthood or religious life" (Suprema Sacra Congregazione del S. Offizio (SSCSO), 1953, p. 1). The book, in their view, did not simply raise disagreeable opinions but jeopardized the holiness of the clergy.

However, while the book was seen as dangerous, Oraison received praise. Geraud argued "the author must be praised first and foremost for his courage. It takes a lot to approach such a vast and complex subject" (1952, p. 6). Geraud, who never met Oraison, suspected he possessed a "dynamic priestly personality" (1952, p. 6). Philippe, who met Oraison a few times, agreed. He described Oraison as "lively, intelligent, [with a] sympathetic mind" (SSCSO, 1953, p. 8) While Oraison seemed to lack "a little restraint in his expressions," Philippe believed him to be "profoundly good and well-oriented" (SSCSO, 1953, p. 8).

There was, therefore, a significant conflict in the review of the book and the author. How could a "profoundly good and well-oriented" man with a "dynamic priestly personality" write with "courage" a book which was "seriously harmful to souls?" It appears the critics saw Oraison as rather naïve and pitiable. Philippe stated, "I suppose (but I do not know) that he must have suffered in his childhood and in his training. This would explain the exaggerations in his book" (SSCSO, 1953, p. 8). Philippe tried his hand in a bit of speculative lay psychoanalysis! That Oraison "must have suffered" is ambiguous enough to be true for anyone, but it does not "explain" anything about the book.

Oraison affirmed the general doctrine of the Church regarding the need for moral sexuality. However, he saw significant problems with the way the Church went about teaching it and responding to those struggling with sexuality. Oraison (1952, p. 51) argued a legalistic approach to sexual morality makes sexuality purely about behavior and whether people are engaging in permitted or forbidden behavior. Sex is then a matter of judicial prudence. A question of legality requires an endless clarification of the law and reduces human sexuality to its most minor movements.

Without an experienced connection between Church morality and lived reality, people "no longer see the reasons for these moral demands, nor the practical means of complying with them" (Oraison, 1952, p. 52). The Church under Pius XII lamented that the world had lost the notion of sin. Yet it did not seem to consider how its teaching contributed to the chasm in which the concept fell out of relevance. Legalism, Oraison (1952, p. 17) argued, "rests on the fundamental notion of repression." Legalism, therefore, is the handmaid of censorship.

Oraison argued legalism implicated the framework of mortal and venial sin. According to the Catechism of the Catholic Church (CCC), mortal sin "destroys charity in the heart of man by a grave violation of God's law...by preferring an inferior good to him" (CCC, 1995, para. 1855). Mortal sin requires the sacrament of reconciliation (confession) to return "sanctifying grace" (CCC, 1995, para. 1861). Venial sin, on the other hand, allows for the continuation of charity. Mortal sin requires "full knowledge and deliberate consent" (CCC, 1995, para. 1857).

Oraison argued that applying a strict behavioral definition to mortal sin again betrays a mere theoretical understanding of life rather than the complexities of reality. He referenced St. Thomas Aquinas to argue how "some sin which is by its nature mortal (particularly grave) becomes venial: namely because the act is imperfect" (Oraison, 1970, p. 61). Such imperfection is the result of a lack of freedom and incomplete consent. With the insights provided by psychoanalysis, the extent to which one can fully know themselves and their acts and whether complete consent is even possible, makes mortal sin "a rare event" (Oraison, 1970, p. 63).

Oraison essentially advocated for a distinction between sin and symptom. The symptom, understood in psychoanalysis as something the patient complains of (Fink, 1997, p. 13), is much more common than mortal sin. Such a "conception of life and salvation...is much more dynamic than legal" (Oraison, 1952, p. 64). Morality is no longer a "statement of sanctions," but a "progressive education from a stage perhaps deeply mired in material sin" (Oraison, 1952, p. 64). Sin is therefore an indication of a necessary area of growth rather than crime for the Church to adjudicate and punish.

Tromp vehemently disagreed. "What the author says about mortal sin cannot be admitted both theoretically and practically" and on this point alone, censorship on the Index was necessary with "danger" in any delay in doing so (SSCSO, 1953, p. 6). For Tromp, Oraison's position called into question the "validity" of the sacraments, particularly marriage and religious life. Geraud (1952, p. 10) agreed. If a person cannot be fully knowledgeable and fully consenting to their marriage or their vocation, then those commitments are invalid.

For Tromp and Geraud, any disorder needed to be resolved prior to the commitment. In the case of priests, Geraud (1952, p. 12) argued "it is not permissible to allow a subject to enter the priesthood who cannot be cured, through the normal path of asceticism and sacramental life, of the sexual disorders he presents upon entering the seminary." The notion of a full cure of what is fundamentally awry in human nature is simply unproven, especially for men in their twenties and thirties.

Oraison (1952, p. 80) argued, "The error of traditional moral teaching on sexuality is to implicitly assume that every human being is in full possession of themselves, and that the pathological, in the broad sense, does not exist." For Oraison, the opposite was true. "There is *only* the pathological, in the broadest sense of the word. This is perhaps the most direct affirmation of human humility that modern science allows us to make" (Oraison, 1952, p. 80). Everyone must recognize their limits in meeting the moral ideals taught by the Church. Because of this universal limit, no one can judge another for their sin or their symptoms. Instead, one must show mercy and help the other construct their next step towards the Kingdom of God.

In the end:

> Christian education must include two complementary and inseparable aspects to remain in conformity with the attitude of Christ: incessant reminder of the moral law in its integrity, and knowledge as complete as possible of the real state of the subject, to help him, starting from his own level, to progress slowly but faithfully in a construction of himself in conformity with the desire of God.
>
> (Oraison, 1952, p. 79)

Oraison highlighted an important tension between eternal redemption and material limits which challenged traditional Catholic moral teaching. Yet he did not seek to resolve this tension but used it to insist on the need for mercy over judgment and sacrifice. While there is universal law, there is also a personal relationship with Christ. There is nothing worth censoring in that conclusion.

Franciscan Sublimation

In the series *The New Pope*, directed by Paolo Sorrentino, the fictional Pope John Paul III (John Malkovic) had a conversation with his advisor, Sophia

(Cécile de France), in which he detailed the dilemma described above between the law and human reality. He spoke to the issue of clerical sexual abuse (Sorrentino et al., 2020).

"For, if we forgive them, they will do it again and if we punish them, we are not practicing Christian charity," said Pope John Paul III. "But is there another way?" asked Sophia. "Man cannot be changed, but he can be diverted," said John Paul III. He continued, "Sick loves cannot be treated, Sofia. You can treat cancer, but not love. One possibility, then, is to shift the object of love" (Sorrentino et al., 2020).

While Sorrentino did not use precise psychoanalytic terms, this description of shifting the object of love is the essence of sublimation. In his essay *On Narcissism*, Freud (1957a, p. 94) defined sublimation as a process which "consists in the instinct's directing itself towards an aim other than, and remote from, that of sexual satisfaction; in this process the accent falls upon deflection from sexuality."

Sophia asked John Paul III, "How do you do that? Tell me!" He replied, "We have to legitimize possible love, so as to divert people from aberrant love, which is a form of violence" (Sorrentino et al., 2020). However, moral law implemented via legalism prohibits and censors possible love rather than providing constructive avenues for its expression.

John Paul III did not advocate for the irrelevance of the moral law. In using the language of aberrant love, and its violence, he recognized an important limit the law needs to perform. Violence as a limit harkens back to Hesnard's focus on the moral consequences of actions. It is not merciful for that violence to occur. But the solution was not repression or censorship, for violence was the result of those processes.

For John Paul III, the shift meant allowing marriage for priests. However, he was "not so naive as to think that this is the solution. But as a way of limiting the damage, it could well work" (Sorrentino et al., 2020). Repression and censorship were not solutions for sexual conflict but neither is sublimation. So why encourage the diversion, why suggest sublimation? It limits the damage. As he put it, "A small step and hopefully less tears in the great ocean of human history." Sublimation is merciful.

Pope Francis insisted on the centrality of Christian mercy. Francis (2016, p. 8) appealed to the etymology of the word when he defined mercy as "opening one's heart to wretchedness." God is the one who opens his heart to wretchedness. Indeed, mercy is "God's identity card" (Francis, 2016, p. 9). An opening up to wretchedness means that mercy requires the exposure rather than the censorship of sin.

"Humanity is wounded, deeply wounded," said Francis (2016, p. 16) and yet people "lack the actual concrete experience of mercy." Legalism is not mercy. Legalism cannot meet people in their concrete existence. "Mostly, people are looking for someone to listen to them. Someone willing to grant them time, to listen to their dramas and difficulties" (Francis, 2016, p. 17).

People want someone to listen, not judge, not censor, and not sanction them. Desire, however aberrant, must be disclosed and heard by another.

The sacrament of reconciliation is where Catholics disclose their sins. Pope Francis (2016, p. 27) insisted that the confessional must not be a "torture chamber." People come to be heard, not "interrogated." How different a perspective and experience compared to that of Marc Oraison being interrogated and silenced in the Holy Office. Legalism interrogates and censors. Mercy listens and blesses.

Pope Francis (2016, p. 66) distinguished between the "logic of the scholars of the law" and the "logic of God." "On the one hand," Francis taught, "there is a fear of losing the just and saved, the sheep that are already safely inside the pen" (Francis, 2016, p. 66). Here is the Holy Office, concerned about "dangerous" texts which would corrupt the souls of the faithful and lead people in religious life to abandon their vocations. "On the other hand, there is the desire to save the sinners, the lost, those on the other side of the fence" (Francis, 2016, p. 66). The logic of God is the desire to save, to show mercy.

The moral law is not the truth. Obedience to the law is not the truth. As Pope Francis (2016, p. 43) taught, "The truth is not grasped as a thing; the truth is encountered. It is not a possession; it is an encounter with a Person." Mercy legitimizes possible love to move people closer to an encounter with truth.

Pope Francis used multiple examples of his encounters with women prostitutes who were simply trying to provide for their families in the midst of extreme poverty. One young woman left the profession to live with a man who was not her husband. After ensuring this man was not taking advantage of the woman, Francis (2016, pp. 72–73) concluded this woman had taken a step towards the truth. While Francis seemed to encourage marriage, he did not condemn her for adultery.

Sublimation is a compromise towards the truth. Sublimation, for Freud (1957a), was one path towards satisfaction of the drives. "The formation of an ideal heightens the demands of the ego and is the most powerful factor favouring repression; sublimation is a way out, a way by which those demands can be met *without* involving repression" (Freud (1957a, p. 95). The formation of an ideal entails a whole domain of desires which are incompatible with the ideal which need to be repressed. Sublimation is a way for desire to be expressed, but towards a different object.

What characterizes the sublimated object? Lacan (1992, p. 94) argued social valor, group approval, and public utility. Sublimation is made possible through objects which hold social value. This social nature of sublimation is what makes sublimation a moral issue. Whereas repression smacks down desire with the judgment, "unacceptable," sublimation works by saying, "unacceptable, but try this act instead." This alternative, nonsexual, behavior is of a higher value. Society values cultural achievements, such as a Picasso painting, rather than people having sex in public.

This transformation from sexual to nonsexual is not quite accurate for Lacan. Sublimation is not a change in aim but a partial satisfaction of the same aim. Sublimation provides satisfaction as a temporary substitute along that aim. Sublimation raises an object to the dignity of the Thing, made in our Image. The Thing is the imagined object which fills the lack which divides the subject. It does not exist in reality but each person is driven to search for it.

Complete sublimation is not possible because there is always something which cannot be sublimated (Lacan, 1992, p. 91). There is a core demand for direct satisfaction that cannot be substituted, displaced, repressed, etc. Therefore, Lacan cautioned against seeing psychoanalysis as a process of normalization. While it might seem better to have sublimated acts to ward off aggressive and sexual instincts, sublimation is not really the goal of analysis. Such a conceptualization is what he referred to as the domain of the pastoral; an idyllic, balanced, harmonic world which will not exist on this side of heaven.

The problem with sublimation is that the moral conscience which is supposed to facilitate it often has the opposite effect. "The moral conscience," wrote Lacan (1992, p. 89),

> shows itself to be the more demanding the more refined it becomes, crueller and crueller even as we offend it less and less, more and more fastidious as we force it, by abstaining from acts, to go and seek out at the most intimate levels of our impulses or desires.

To consider the Christian tradition, as Lacan did, Jesus gave two great commandments. One look at current Canon Law shows how greatly expanded, and demanding, the Church has become.

People can never be ethical enough for their consciences. There is always a standard yet to be met. If an individual has cleared the low bars of what it means to be a civilized person, the rules narrow. Why? Sublimation, even though it is a way of trying to satisfy the drive, is doing so via a surrogate object, and in this way, fundamentally opposes the drive. Sublimation is still not giving the drive what it truly wants.

That is why Lacan (1992, p. 95) wrote, "Freud is telling us the same thing as Saint Paul," that there is no Sovereign Good. There is no essential ethical rule an individual can grasp for complete satisfaction or complete elimination of guilt. People are in a constant process of interrogating the good or pleasure they are seeking and must justify why they want it. Sublimation, like repression, requires constant maintenance. Yet sublimation at least allows for the expression of desire, however diverted or substituted.

Jesus was asked, "What good must I do to achieve eternal life?" and he replied, "Why do you speak to me of good?" (Matt. 19:16–17). There is no good which we can know and possess to guarantee salvation, we only have commandments to follow (Lacan, 1992, p. 96). Jesus listed various commandments and ended with love your neighbor as yourself. The constructive, not prohibitive, moral law is summed up in the command to show mercy. Sublimation, while narcissistic in its appeal to the object for personal satisfaction, is also selfless in the sense that the object becomes something of value to society, not just the individual.

Jorge in *The Name of the Rose* and the Holy Office contra Hesnard and Oraison idealized and identified themselves with the object (law) and enacted censorship and repression to achieve it. Sublimation via Pope Francis and Lacan, on the other hand, recognizes and welcomes desire. In contrast with Freud's superego guard in his drawing room, Christianity offers the father waiting at the door to welcome the prodigal son.

Psychoanalysis is a small step towards the truth. Like the fictional John Paul III, Lacan did not see his aim as cure. Evans (1996, p. 55) summarized Lacan's position thus:

> The end of analysis is not the disappearance of the symptom, nor the cure of an underlying disease (for example, neurosis), since analysis is not essentially a therapeutic process but a search for the truth, and the truth is not always beneficial.

For Pope Francis, the sacramental life was not about the disappearance of sin nor the cure of original sin but a search for *the* Truth, an encounter with Jesus.

Merciful sublimation does not produce a completely healthy individual, but someone oriented towards the truth of their unconscious and of God. As Lacan wrote, "[psychoanalysis] makes possible a cure in which the subject is not alienated from himself, and the responsibility it restores in him responds to the hope, which throbs in every hated being, of integrating himself into a lived meaning" ("Discussion des Rapports," 1951, p. 88). Mercy stands at the door of the consulting room and welcomes the suffering patient to work towards this lived meaning.

References

Barbierato, F. (2022). Index of prohibited books. In M. Sgarbi (Ed.), *Encyclopedia of Renaissance philosophy* (pp. 1670–1676). Springer.

Catechism of the Catholic Church: with modifications from the Editio Typica (CCC). (1995). Revised in accordance with the official Latin text promulgated by Pope John Paul II. Doubleday.

Discussion des rapports. (1951). *Revue Français de Psychanalyse*, 15(1): 62–88.

Eco, U. (2023). *The name of the rose*. (W. Weaver, Trans.). Harper.

Evans, D. (1996). *An introductory dictionary of Lacanian psychoanalysis*. Routledge.

Fink, B. (1997). *A clinical introduction to Lacanian psychoanalysis: theory and technique*. Harvard University Press.

Francis (2016). *The name of God is mercy*. Random House.

Freud, S. (1957a). On narcissism. In J. Strachey (Ed. & Trans.), *The standard edition of the complete psychological works of Sigmund Freud*, Vol. 14 (pp. 67–116). Hogarth Press. (Original work published 1914)

Freud, S. (1957b). Repression. In J. Strachey (Ed. & Trans.), *The standard edition of the complete psychological works of Sigmund Freud*, Vol. 14 (pp. 141–158). Hogarth Press. (Original work published 1915)

Freud, S. (1961). Civilization and its discontents. In J. Strachey (Ed. & Trans.), *The standard edition of the complete psychological works of Sigmund Freud*, Vol. 21 (pp. 57–146). Hogarth Press. (Original work published 1930)

Gemelli, A. (1955). "Morale sans péché": Une étude du R.P. Gemelli sur un livre récent. Secrétariat de L'Episcopat. *Archives of the Dicastery for the Doctrine of the Faith*. Note 37/55. Vatican.

Geraud, J. (1952). Notes de psychiatrie et recension de "vie chretienne et problémes de la sexualité" de Marc Oraison. Archives of the Dicastery for the Doctrine of the Faith. C.L. 388_1952/i. Vatican.

Hesnard, A. (1949). *L'univers morbide de la faute*. Presses Universitaires de France.

Hesnard, A. (1954). *Morale sans péché*. Presses Universitaires de France.

Lacan, J. (1992). *Book VII: The ethics of psychoanalysis: 1959–1960*. (D. Porter, Trans.). W.W. Norton & Company.

Laplanche, J. & Pontalis, J.B. (1973). *The language of psycho-analysis*. W.W. Norton & Company.

Oraison, M. (1952). *Vie chretienne et problémes de la sexualité*. P. Lethielleux.

Oraison, M. (1970). *Strange voyage: The autobiography of a nonconformist*. Doubleday.

Philippe, P. (1954). Francia-Parigi: Dr. A. Hesnard, "Morale sans péché": Nota della cancelleria. Suprema Sacra Congregazione del S. Offizio. Prot. Num. 353/54/i. Vatican.

Philippe, P. (1955). Francia-Parigi: Libri del Dr. A. Hesnard: Breve relazione pro secreta. Suprema Sacra Congregazione del S. Offizio. Prot. S.O. 353/54/i. Vatican.

Pius XII (1953). *Speech by Pope Pius XII to participants in the international congress of psychotherapy and clinical psychology*. https://www.papalencyclicals.net/pius12/p12psyre.htm.

Plé, A. (1980). *Duty or pleasure? A new appraisal of Christian ethics*. Paragon House Publishers.

Ricoeur, P. (1955). "Morality without sin" or sin without moralism? *CrossCurrents*, 5(4): 339–352.

Sorrentino, P. (Writer & Director), Contarello, U. (Writer), & Bises, S. (Writer). (2020, January 24). Season 1, Episode 5. [TV Series episode]. In L. Mieli, M. Gianani, R. Neri, E. Recchia, P. Sorrentino, J. Law, C. Benjo, C. Scotta, S. Arnal, J. Roures, J. Méndez, N. Hartmann, S. Rovai, & D. Bertoni (Executive Producers). *The New Pope*. The Apartment Pictures; Wildside; Haut et Court TV; Mediapro; Sky Studios.

Suprema Sacra Congregazione del S. Offizio (SSCSO). (1953). Intorno al libro: "Vie Chrétienne et problémes de la sexualité." Prot. 388/52/i. Archivio del Dicastero per la Dottrina della Fede. Vatican City.

Vose, R. (2022). *The index of prohibited books: Four centuries of struggle over word and image for the greater glory of God*. Reaktion Books.

Winfield, N. (2013, July 29). "Who am I to judge?" pope says of gay priests. Associated Press News. https://apnews.com/general-news-7b465b60945f40deb3a68b3de742f84a.

Chapter 5

Ressourcement and Original Sin

Rahner with Lacan

Ressourcement theology was a method of scholarship and spiritual revival which emerged in the 1930s–1950s among Jesuits in France and spread to other countries like Germany in the 1960s. This method employed a "return to the sources" of Christian tradition, doctrine, and practice to interrogate and develop solutions for contemporary problems in the Church and the world (Boersma, 2009). Though significant differences existed among these theologians, the term *nouvelle theologie* or new theology was used by Charles Boyer (1940) and Monsignor Pietro Parente (1942) to group them together for the purpose of heated criticism.

Pius XII saw the "new theologians" as a threat to Neo-Scholasticism which was the theological/philosophical foundation for the teaching of the Magisterium in the decade following the First Vatican Council (Del Colle, 2010). The Church felt compelled to respond to the promotion of reason in the European Enlightenment (seventeenth and eighteenth centuries) and the anticlericalism and anti-Catholicism of the French Revolution (eighteenth century).

The Church needed to clarify its theology to counter the charge that faith was opposed to reason while also retaining the supernatural basis of faith. As Del Colle (2010, p. 375) argued, "Neo-Scholastic theology and philosophy were part of a diverse Catholic theological endeavor to adjudicate the intellectual foundations and interpretation of faith amid the emerging culture of Western modernity." The Church sought to integrate the philosophy of the enlightenment (particularly Immanuel Kant) in its elaboration of reason while also sustaining the "intelligibility of faith" (through Thomas Aquinas) (Del Colle, 2010, p. 378).

Pope Leo XIII's (1879) encyclical *Aeterni Patris* was "responding to the contemporary problem of how faith and reason needed to be integrated to enable an adequate and comprehensive response to the contestation over truth and religion" (Del Colle, 2010, p. 376). How to determine what is true was a central problem for secular philosophy as society moved away from the pure divine revelation the Church taught as the method of truth.

The question of truth was not only a question of cognitive knowledge but also of the lived experience of the body. The tension between faith and reason was, therefore, closely related to the relationship between divine grace and human

DOI: 10.4324/9781003485346-7

nature. What is the truth of the nature of being human? As this chapter will show, original sin is a doctrine that is directly implicated in this relationship.

Unfortunately, as Del Colle (2010, p. 382) outlined, what was meant to be a wider engagement in disciplines outside the Church was instead a conflict "within the Church contesting against existing Catholic efforts in this arena." This insular conflict continued into the papacy of Pius XII. The papal endorsement of genuine interdisciplinary dialogue morphed into a narrow reading of Thomas Aquinas which produced unquestionable theological treatises and doctrines. In other words, Neo-Scholasticism experienced a similar calcification to the theology it attempted to liven in the first place. Neo-Scholastic theologians came to stand in opposition to the world rather than engage with it.

This calcification of doctrine, rather than specific ideas themselves, was the target of *ressourcement* theology. These theologians saw Neo-Scholasticism as ahistorical, that is, it paid no attention to real human events. Rather than show how the mystery of God is intimately relevant to the problems of everyday life, neo-scholastic theology offered theoretical syllogisms to "prove" the truthfulness of Christianity (D'Ambrosio, 1991). Truly collaborative, dynamic dialogue was therefore a threat to what Pius XII (1950) referred to as the "immanent," "immutable," and "absolute" doctrine of the Church. Combined with the Neo-Scholastic introduction of papal infallibility through the First Vatican Council, to question the Magisterium and the pope was to question God.

Criticism of Modernism, with its emphasis on subjective experience through empiricism and its rejection of traditionalism, was a refrain for Pius XII. He made his position on Modernism clear in his encyclical *Humani Generis* (1950), criticizing the theory of evolution (paras. 5–6), the philosophy of existentialism (para. 6), and the practice of historicism (para. 7). He then warned of how the new theologians' engagement with modernism threatened longstanding Catholic truth. Pius XII (1950, para. 34) wrote, "these new opinions endanger the two philosophical sciences which by their very nature are closely connected with the doctrine of faith, that is, theodicy and ethics." Pius XII was right to identify these two topics as major areas of concern for the theologians, but wrong in his conclusion of danger.

The *ressourcement* theologians were not threatened by Modernism. They did not engage in trench apologetics. Instead,

> their goal was to break the 'fortress mentality' and compel Catholic theology to engage in a critical dialogue with twentieth-century thinkers, a dialogue that would send theologians back to the sources with new questions, provoking the rediscovery of forgotten or neglected dimensions of the tradition.
>
> (D'Ambrosio, 1991, p. 549)

Sigmund Freud's publication of *The Interpretation of Dreams* in 1900 established psychoanalysis as a major voice in this regard.

The critics of *ressourcement* saw something shared between *ressourcement* and psychoanalysis. Though the connection between these movements was the result of opposition, there are important insights to be gained in reading this theology alongside psychoanalytic theory. This chapter elaborates this connection through putting into dialogue one of *ressourcement*'s key theologians, Karl Rahner, with one of his contemporaries in psychoanalysis, Jacques Lacan.

One of the problems Pius XII identified, and both Rahner and Lacan approached, albeit with different language and within different contexts, was the question of ethics. People approached priests and psychoanalysts with questions about how to live without suffering. Both Rahner and Lacan recognized the pervasive sense of guilt at the core of this suffering. Rahner reconceptualized the doctrines of original sin and redemption and Lacan reconceptualized the experience of guilt and the goal of psychoanalysis. Both thinkers argued spiritual and psychological freedom, respectively, are the foundation of an ethical life.

Karl Rahner (1904–1984) was a Jesuit priest and a significant figure during the debates of the Second Vatican Council, in the drafting of the official documents, and in their interpretation in the decades that followed the Council. Rahner and the new theologians did not want to reject or elevate tradition. Instead, they wished to return to the sources of tradition and doctrine and explore the possibilities which had been missed for understanding contemporary humanity and God. This desire to return and rethink theology was condemned by Pope Pius XII. But Rahner and his colleagues were highly valued and encouraged by Pope John XXIII as he opened the Second Vatican Council. Rahner and his colleagues argued *ressourcement* was a necessary step towards achieving the *aggiornamento* (accompaniment) which emerged from the Second Vatican Council.

Rahner, later in his career, compiled his decades of scholarship into a tome titled *Foundations of Christian Faith* (1982). This chapter examines Rahner's conceptualization of original sin, its relationship to guilt, and the freedom that Christianity sees at the heart of what it means to be human. But why Rahner? With psychoanalysis at its peak during the decade surrounding Vatican II, and many theologians and priests actively dialoguing with psychoanalysts, it does not seem Rahner ever directly engaged with psychoanalysis. Yet a few aspects are relevant to psychoanalysis.

First, the French word associated with the new theologians – *ressourcement* – parallels Jacques Lacan's famous "return to Freud," or, one could say, return to the sources of psychoanalysis to rethink psychoanalytic theory and practice. Whereas the new theologians understood Neo-Scholasticism as drifting far from its origin in Thomas Aquinas, Lacan (2013), p. 203) argued psychoanalysis had "left fallow" the richness of Freud's teaching regarding the function of language and speech.

But for theologians like Rahner and analysts like Lacan, the solution was not to simply restate historical documents but to use history as a resource to address the new problems of contemporary life. There was a similar project between Rahner and Lacan in this regard. *Ressourcement* is not just a method of scholarship for theology or psychoanalysis, but also the method of confession and psychoanalysis. Psychoanalysts and priests return to the sources of symptoms and sins to develop new ways of living.

Second, Rahner's (1982) third chapter is titled, "Man as a Being Threatened Radically by Guilt." If one did not know the context, this title could easily come from an article in a psychoanalytic journal. Rahner understood guilt as an essential component of human nature. Rahner recognized the experience of guilt for modern people does not stem from a fear of God, as in centuries past. Nevertheless, guilt affects them, but they cannot name it as such. For Rahner (1982, p. 105), the threat of guilt is "really a permanent existential which we can never eradicate in our single, temporal history."

The centrality of guilt in understanding the struggles of humanity parallels Lacan's (and Freud's) understanding of unconscious, primordial guilt. The unconscious, where guilt is situated, is not something which can be eradicated in the psyche of an individual but is, in the words of Rahner, an "existential" given in human life. The goal cannot be eradication, but a changed relationship to the existential.

Third, Rahner's idea of a fundamental option, the human capacity to say no to God, insists on a choice that must be made by every person. This potential no to God is also a denial of what it means to be human, made in the image of God. To say no is therefore a rejection of human freedom made possible by God. To say no to God is also a rejection of self-knowledge. This is why Rahner (1982, p. 97) referred to this choice as the freedom to "dispose of oneself." Human subjectivity is ontologically and eschatologically tied to God.

For Lacan, this choice can only freely be made once one has confronted their unconscious desire(s). A person cannot freely choose God if they are repressing, disavowing, or foreclosing on their desires. Yet this freedom exists parallel to guilt and collective and individual original sin.

Why Lacan? There are, after all, other psychoanalysts who personally share the faith of the Catholic Church and have written about this intersection before and after Lacan. Lacan clearly split from Freud in the latter's often harsh and personal attacks on religious belief, particularly Catholicism. Lacan valued Catholic thinkers and theology as evidenced by those in his institutional circles, such as Maryse Choisy, Michel de Certeau, Angelo Hesnard, and Antoine Vergote, some condemned by the Vatican. Like Rahner and the *ressourcement* theologians, Lacan (2007, p. 204) criticized in his own discipline the "ahistoricism" which is "diametrically opposed to analytic experience." Personal and collective history matters.

This chapter draws from the seventh year of Lacan's (1986) seminars, between 1959–1960, when he taught on the ethics of psychoanalysis. It was during this academic year Lacan was invited to give a lecture to the Catholic

University of Leuven. Lacan's primary contribution to the ongoing dialogue with Catholic theology was his conceptualization of unconscious desire which he articulated in his formal seminar in Paris and the lecture in Belgium.

Rahner's understanding of guilt combined with Lacan's understanding of desire offers an integration of theory and theology regarding what it means for people to possess and exercise spiritual and psychological freedom. First is a review of Rahner's definitions of guilt and original sin. Then Lacan's conceptualization of unconscious desire is explicated within the context of Rahner's work. In the end, this chapter practices *ressourcement* to gain a fresh understanding of the relevance of original sin for contemporary society and psychoanalytic practice.

Rahner on Guilt and Original Sin

Rahner stated guilt and sin are central to Christianity because Christianity is a story of redemption from guilt and sin. Rahner (1982, p. 90) used an interesting word alongside guilt – "forlornness" – to describe the unhappiness or dissatisfaction humanity experiences because of sin. Forlornness suggests a sense of loss, of being alone, and, consequently, of longing for something to resolve that loss. Rahner's use of forlornness echoes the Lacanian notion of lack, which will be discussed further below.

Another tenet of Christianity is that humanity cannot through its own means resolve this dissatisfaction. Rahner understood many people today would not describe their life experience in this way. He wrote the question of justification before God "does not bother people today very much or maybe even not at all" (Rahner, 1982, p. 91). He attributed this lack of awareness in part to the social sciences. "The modern social sciences have a thousand ways and means to 'unmask' the experience of man's guilt before God and to demolish it as a false taboo" (Rahner, 1982, p. 91).

In psychoanalysis, however, there is no such thing as a *false* taboo, and Lacan had no interest in unmasking or absolving the experience of guilt in his patients. Guilt surely bothers contemporary people, but it is often not spiritual or conscious. Guilt for most people today is unconscious. People look to justify themselves, but not before God, but before those with whom they identify in their everyday life.

Rahner recognized that while people may be able to remain unaware of their position before God, they are aware of their position before one another. In other words, there remains secular morality. Rahner (1982, p. 91) wrote, "It cannot be denied that man is responsible, that he is accountable, that...he has the experience of being able to come and of actually coming into conflict with himself and his original self-understanding." This remark of coming into conflict with oneself and self-understanding should perk the ears of any psychoanalyst. As Rahner (1982, p. 91) wryly described, denying this conflict only "plunges people into neurotic anxiety." Of course, for psychoanalysts, neurotic anxiety is defined by this internal conflict with oneself. In Lacanian terminology, Rahner simply described the split subject.

Rahner argued whether people use a Christian/religious framework or a secular one, humans are moral beings. The conflict, as Rahner saw it, was between who a person should be and who they are now. Yet original sin as an existential truth has fallen out of favor in secular Western society. Rather than people having to justify their sins, and the negative consequences of those sins in the world to God, humanity asks God to justify himself to them about theodicy. "Why does God allow bad things to happen?" is the prototypical question in this regard. At the extreme, death is seen not as a consequence of sin but the resolution of the absurdity of existence. Rahner argued guilt can only be understood within the Christian framework of justification and redemption. Guilt, as Rahner (1982, p. 93) defined it, is the "closing oneself to the offer of God's absolute self-communication." He went on, "It is only in the process of forgiveness to which a person opens himself and accepts that he can understand what the guilt is that is being forgiven" (Rahner, 1982, p. 93). In other words, only when believing in the loving and forgiving God can one understand the seriousness of their guilt.

As the Catholic philosopher and psychoanalyst Antoine Vergote (1988), of the University of Leuven, once wrote, "The promise of salvation implies that a wound inflicted upon man and society has diminished and demeaned them both," and that wound is called sin. Yet, "biblical thought does not locate these forces in the cosmos, nor in the body, nor in the passions," it is, within scripture, a mystery (Vergote, 1988, p. 43). Psychoanalysis locates these forces within the unconscious.

This belief or lack thereof regarding guilt and sin speaks to human freedom. To be free, Rahner wrote, is to be responsible for ourselves. Freedom is the wholeness of existence, the "capacity of the one subject to decide about himself in his single totality" (Rahner, 1982, p. 94). Rahner was not talking about freedom in the political sense, of a series of rights to speak or assemble. Freedom is an act of subjectivity. It is the freedom to self-actualize in a way that cannot be undone. Rahner (1982, p. 96) wrote, "wherever there is no freedom, there is always just something which by its nature goes on generating itself and becoming something else and being reduced to something else." Freedom is opposed to the psychoanalytic notion of repetition compulsion. Repetition compulsion is being stuck in the past of who one once was whereas freedom is the capacity to and experience of change.

This freedom, however, is conditioned by the limits of this world. One may act and live within their freedom, but the world is something else. Through everyday life, people are constantly asked the question of their freedom. Even when people choose to say yes to this freedom and the God at its horizon, Rahner (1982, p. 98) taught we are merely affirming the God of "thematic, categorical reflection, to a God in concepts, maybe even only to a God in false gods." In Lacanian terms, people cannot affirm a God in the register of the Real, for that God is unknowable and literally unspeakable, but only God in Symbolic and Imaginary ways, with the words and images available and which necessarily limit human understanding.

Rahner (1982, p. 100) taught "freedom is the freedom to say 'yes' or 'no' to God, and therein and thereby it is freedom in relation to oneself." Saying yes or no to God is saying yes or no to our self, a validation or a denial of our self. But yes and no, while they are two possible responses, are not equal responses. Yes is an eternal yes, but no is in theory never absolute, because the possibility of saying no is only "intelligible" in comparison to the yes. There remains the mystery of evil, but while we have an eschatology of heaven, hell is much murkier. Hell on earth is the appropriate phrase to describe those who attempt such a definitive, evil, no in this life. How life on this planet will end, collectively and individually, is always unknown. Regardless, there remains a choice. Rahner (1982, p. 104) said, "In and through yourself, in and through what you in your innermost depths are and definitively want to be, you can be a person who closes himself into the absolute, deadly and final loneliness of saying 'no' to God."

Returning to Vergote (1988, p. 4), he wrote, "freedom is entrenched in the body and in the unconscious." He used the example of demon possession, and the idea that personal transgression was linked to its etiology. While rightly dismissive of the causality characteristic of the Middle Ages, Vergote (1988, p. 4) argued "an interpretation that regards the possessed as responsible agents at least does not treat their disorders as byproducts of a mechanical body but rather links mental alienation to a personal history." This link between mental alienation and personal history is both Catholic and psychoanalytic, both spiritual and psychical.

The possibility of no to God is intimately related to the possibility for sin. Rahner (1982, p. 104) argued the possibility of sin is a permanent existential which "cannot be eradicated." He described people as free subjects who are constantly threatened by themselves. "This threat is really a permanent existential which we can never eradicate in our single, temporal history" (Rahner, 1982, p. 105). This is a struggle which all people will experience until death. This struggle is not pathological, or at least, it is a pathology which afflicts all people. This closely relates to Lacan's structures of the mind, diagnoses of neurosis, perversion, and psychosis, which everyone falls into in a way that is sharply differentiated from the psychopathology in the DSM. Human existence is structured by this struggle, by the internal conflict between what we are and what we want to become.

Overwhelmingly, Catholic theologians argue one cannot speak of sin without speaking also of redemption. Analogous to psychoanalysis, one cannot speak of diagnosis without speaking also of treatment. For Lacan, proper diagnosis is important because it orients the psychoanalyst to the approach needed for the patient. For priests, a proper conceptualization of sin is important insofar as it orients their work with their parishioners. In both cases, a pure focus on behavior is not sufficient for the needs of humanity.

Original sin is part of what it means to be human. It is the condition that both confirms birth and death. The Garden of Eden was an experience of the Real, where Adam and Eve walked with God without any Symbolic or Imaginary mediation (literal clothing and divine masking). Humanity cannot return to that origin, if it ever existed in history, but is stuck within the limits of the Symbolic and Imaginary registers. As Rahner (1982, p. 106) wrote, "We have neither the possibility nor the right to give back our admission ticket to existence, a ticket which is still used and not allowed to expire even when someone tries to annihilate himself in a suicide attempt." We must spend the ticket; we cannot trash it or transfer it or sell it. This is the contingency of freedom. The freedom to choose, and we must choose.

Rahner (1982, p. 107) acknowledged the pre-existing world into which humans are born, "imposed on him, and which is ultimately the presupposition of his freedom…he actualizes himself as a free subject in a situation which itself is always determined by history and by other persons." What Rahner described here is aligned with what Lacan termed the Symbolic register of existence, the history, people, language, and cultural norms which structure, limit, and direct daily life and self-understanding. Human freedom is influenced by how others have exercised their freedom.

Consequently, personal guilt is influenced by how others have experienced and coped with their guilt. This co-determination of the situation by the guilt of others is "something universal, permanent, and therefore also original" (Rahner, 1982, p. 109). Universal in the sense that everyone shares it, permanent in that it is with us until death, and original, "that is, already imbedded in the origin of this history to the extent that this origin of the single history of the human race is to be understood as established by man" (Rahner, 1982, p. 110). Sin is original in the sense that it began with human action, not with God.

This understanding of original sin is contrary to the idea of Adam's sin extending to contemporary people. As Rahner (1982, p. 110) taught:

> The notion that the personal deed of 'Adam' or the of the first group of people is imputed to us in such a way that is has been transmitted on to us biologically, as it were, has absolutely nothing to do with the Christian dogma of original sin.

Original sin is human sin, co-determined by the tension between guilt and freedom experienced throughout human history up until the present and its possibility in the future.

As the Jesuit Father Peter Dempsey (1951, p. 491) argued, while baptism removes the barrier between the individual and God, "psychologically, subjectively – *quoad nos* – the tendency towards guilt remains, because the disorder and the defect remain." The world is presently disordered, and each human born into the world is psychologically affected by it. Original sin, while spiritually configured, exerts its effects on the human psyche. As Rahner

(1982, p. 110) argued, we come to understand original sin through a "religious-existential interpretation of our own situation, from ourselves." There is a collective experience of original sin but a personal recognition of guilt and the choice that must be made to engage with this guilt. Rahner wrote, "Personal guilt from an original act of freedom cannot be transmitted, for it is the *existentiell* 'no' of personal transcendence towards God or against him." (Rahner, 1982, p. 111). There is original sin as the structure of human experience after Eden and there is personal sin in the choices everyone makes in their life.

Rahner argued not only does contemporary man not inherit original sin from Adam, but the story of the first sin is rather a logical deduction and explanation of our experience of sin in the present.

> The portrayal of the sin of the first man is rather an etiological inference from the experience of man's existential situation in the history of salvation to what must have happened 'at the beginning' if the present situation of freedom actually is the way it is experienced, and if it is accepted as it is.
>
> (Rahner, 1982, p. 114)

Humanity does not inherit sin from a historical Adam, but mythological Adam is conceived from the real experiences of humanity. For whoever wrote the stories of Genesis 1–3, it was their own experience of sin and guilt which led them to imagine its origin through this story.

By not seeing this beginning as rigidly historical, "God's self-communication in grace comes to man not from 'Adam,' not from the beginning of the human race, but from the goal of this history, from the God-Man Jesus Christ" (Rahner, 1982, p. 114). For Rahner, the conceptualization of original sin is directed at the future, not the past.

This reversal in the directionality of original sin is like the way Freud inferred and narrated the myth of the primal horde and the murder of the father as the origin of the Oedipus Complex, discussed below. How one conceives of guilt and sin in the present makes a difference for how a better future is to be achieved.

Humanity's future is not determined by Adam's behavior but by the freedom each person must exercise in their relationship with God. Similarly, the neurotic patient's psyche in psychoanalysis is not causally determined by their childhood, but by the choices they make in the present and future, about whether to acknowledge or repress their unconscious desire.

In summary, Rahner viewed guilt and sin as central to Christianity, framing them as the foundation of humanity's need for redemption. He used the concept of "forlornness" to describe the dissatisfaction and longing people feel due to sin, a sense of loss that humanity cannot resolve through its own means. While modern individuals may not be conscious of their guilt before

God, they are aware of their moral conflict with themselves and others. Rahner emphasized that guilt can only be understood through a Christian lens of justification and redemption, and freedom is the capacity to choose one's relationship with God. He argued original sin is not inherited from Adam but is an existential experience rooted in human freedom, shaping both personal sin and collective guilt. For Rahner, the future of humanity is determined not by past actions but by the individual's freedom to choose their path toward God.

Lacan on Guilt and Desire

Lacan oriented his discussion on ethics around the choices people make regarding the limits provided to them, both external in terms of societal law and internal in terms of internalized law. To engage in something unethical, one transgresses a limit. This term – transgression – is important. Lacan referenced work on transgression by Hesnard, referenced in chapter four, a fellow French psychoanalyst, and founding member of Lacan's institute, the SPP. Hesnard's book *Morality without Sin* was censored by the Vatican and placed on their infamous Index of Prohibited Books.

Ethics is not only about right and wrong but the attraction of the unethical, the appeal of transgression. The act of transgression is not simply about the moral law. People make choices about how to act with a direction in mind. Obedience or transgression entails a trajectory towards an image of goodness. And the actions which people take – or don't take – through obedience or transgression to reach that Imaginary goodness have consequences. Lacan argued the primary consequence of not taking steps towards one's desired Good – which he saw time and again in his clinical practice – is guilt.

Lacan's conceptualization of desire should be understood as an aspect of freedom described by Rahner. After all, freedom is the capacity to make a choice, and we make choices based on what we desire. What connects desire to guilt? Lacan referred to Freud's (1913) myth of the primordial horde in *Totem and Taboo* which underpinned his concept of the Oedipal Complex. "Guilt finds its roots at the unconscious level, where it is linked to a fundamental crime for which no one can individually answer, nor has to" (Lacan, 2005, p. 30). This fundamental crime is the murder of the father of the horde by his sons, for the purpose of gaining access to the mother.

This Freudian myth of the origin of guilt performs a similar function to the Genesis myth of original sin. Freud's pseudo-historical myth is worth reviewing here to see how he retroactively located the origin of the contemporary experience of neurotic guilt. The myth is found in the fifth section of the fourth chapter of *Totem and Taboo*, "The Return of Totemism in Childhood" (Freud, 1913, pp. 140–145). Transgression is at the heart of both stories. Freud took as his starting point the primal horde hypothesized by Darwin.

But this proposal was insufficient for the theoretical complexities Freud attempted to explain. "All that we find there is a violent and jealous father who keeps all the females for himself and drives away his sons as they grow up" (Freud, 1913, p. 140). Here is an original command: sons are forbidden to possess the women belonging to their father.

Freud (1913, p. 140) noted primitive organizations were observed which "consist[ed] of bands of males; these bands are composed of members with equal rights and are subject to the restrictions of the totemic system, including inheritance through the mother." Freud wondered, in retrospect, how such organizations of people came to be. Thus, his myth. Freud (1913, p. 140) wrote:

> One day the brothers who had been driven out [by the father] came together, killed and devoured their father and so made an end of the patriarchal horde...United, they had the courage to do and succeeded in doing what would have been impossible for them individually.

Important for theological innovations emerging from *ressourcement* regarding original sin, this patricide was a collective act. Universal guilt stems from universal sin. Freud (1913, p. 141) continued:

> Cannibal savages as they were, it goes without saying that they devoured their victim as well as killing him. The violent primal father had doubtless been the feared and envied model of each one of the company of brothers: and in the act of devouring him they accomplished their identification with him, and each one of them acquired a portion of his strength. The totem meal, which is perhaps mankind's earliest festival, would thus be a repetition and a commemoration of this memorable and criminal deed, which was the beginning of so many things – of social organization, of moral restrictions and of religion.

The sons' identification with the primal father is preceded by the solidarity each of the sons displayed with one another in the murder. As Kertelge (1991) argued in his commentary on Romans 5:12–21, with the transmission of sin from Adam to his descendants, there is a "corporate personality" at work in the horde. The "original father of a group determines the destiny of his descendants as well" (Kertelge, 1991, p. 509).

Original sin is "not simply fate" but shared history in that people "cannot eliminate themselves from solidarity with all human beings...they positively confirm this solidarity by their own transgression" (Kertelge, 1991, p. 512). Original sin is part of the human condition through the continued, repeated solidarity of humanity demonstrated by individual sin.

Wiedenhofer (1991, p. 518) used Jungian language when he described original sin as "the archetype of sin's nature." To pursue a historical beginning to the archetype of the Joker is as futile as attempting to geographically locate

Eden. Yet the substance and pattern of the Joker is familiar across time and culture. The same is true with original sin. But where is the guilt? Freud (1913, p. 143, emphasis added) continued:

> [We] need only suppose that the tumultuous mob of brothers were filled with the same contradictory feelings which we can see at work in the ambivalent father-complexes of our children and of our neurotic patients. They hated their father, who presented such a formidable obstacle to their craving for power and their sexual desires; but they loved and admired him too.
>
> After they had got rid of him, had satisfied their hatred and had put into effect their wish to identify themselves with him, the affection which had all this time been pushed under was bound to make itself felt. It did so in the form of remorse. *A sense of guilt made its appearance*, which in this instance *coincided with the remorse felt by the whole group.*

One of Freud's basic tenets is that love and hate are inseparable. Where one loves, one also hates. When hate dominated the horde, love was repressed among them. When their hatred was satisfied through murder, love made itself felt. Freud argued guilt was the expression of love following the satisfaction of hate. In summary, desire for the mother led the sons to murder their father, and the guilt about this murder of the father whom they loved led the sons to create the phobic object. This phobic object – representative of the dead father – created distance between the horde and the object of their desire (Freud, 1913, pp. 132–146). In other words, guilt prompted the creation of the moral law.

Lacan took a different approach to understanding guilt. For Lacan, guilt is not about regretting what has already been done, it is about not doing what was ultimately desired. After all, the sons in Freud's myth could not literally become their own father and possess their mother as their wife. Freud (1913, p. 142) admitted as much: "Not one of the sons had in fact been able to put his original wish – of taking his father's place – into effect. And, as we know, failure is far more propitious for a moral reaction than satisfaction." Guilt stemming from original sin, then, is not about having eaten the apple. The guilt we carry from original sin is the failure to be more than human; omnipotent and omniscient.

After Lacan, there were spirited debates between Catholic psychologists on how to interpret the notion of original sin with Freudian psychoanalysis. Their question regarded how original sin presents in the psyche. For Vitz and Gartner (1989), the Oedipus complex was the best representation of original sin. Because he was born without original sin, Jesus was the anti-Oedipus. For Bridgman and Carter (1989), original sin was a preoedipal experience best understood as primary narcissism. Jesus was, then, the non-narcissist. But these positions are staked within a debate framed by fitting the concept of original sin within an existing psychoanalytic concept. What Lacan attempted, and what this chapter follows, is different. Rather than explain one concept by another, Lacan's teaching situates unconscious guilt as preceding original sin. Rahner's theology and Lacan's theory are complementary, not explanatory, of one another.

For Rahner, guilt is both historical and personal, in other words, personal history. Rahner, as quoted above, argued guilt is an *existentiell* of human experience. But Rahner did not examine the phenomenon prior to the act of eating the apple. Catholic theology does not focus on desire as an *existentiell*. Desire, Lacan taught, is the desire of the Other, which is a way of saying what people want has been influenced and conditioned by their families and cultures. One's desire is the result of identification with another's desire.

In the same way in which modern people experience original sin through identification and solidarity with mythical Adam, people today also experience an original desire as an identification. Subjects are split between what they want and what they think they ought to want limited within the context of their history and their future possibilities. Original desire was the precondition for original sin.

In Freudian terms, this split is the tension between the pleasure and reality principles. In Lacanian terms, this split is between unconscious desire and conscious intention. In Catholic theology as outlined by Rahner, this split is between human freedom and original sin. This existential experience is what Lacan referred to as the Split Subject.

Lacan was absolutely opposed to the idea that the development of self-control can address this split. He criticized ego psychology as an example of a broader effort to socialize and tame the ego. In *Discourse to Catholics*, Lacan (2005, p. 9) described the following:

> The ego, considered to be a function both of synthesis and of integration; consciousness, considered to be the culmination of life; evolution considered to be the pathway by which the evolution of consciousness comes into being; the categorical application of this postulate to the individual's psychological development; and the notion of behavior, which is applied in a unitary fashion in order to break every bit of dramatic tension in human life down to the most ridiculous degree.
>
> All of this camouflages the following: nothing in the concrete life of a single individual allows us to ground the idea that such a finality directs his life and could lead him – through the pathways of progressive self-consciousness undergirded by natural development – to harmony with himself as well as to approval from the world on which his happiness depends.

Lacan argued neither the integration of the ego, nor conscious intention, nor behavioral analysis leads to harmony with oneself. What happens in the pursuit of harmony and happiness is that:

> man is ever more impotent to meet up anew with his own desire…this man no longer knows how to find the object of his desire and no longer encounters anything but unhappiness in his search, living in an anguish that progressively shrinks what one might call his change to invent.
>
> (Lacan, 2005, p. 10)

Lacan identified the forlornness Rahner described as the consequence of original sin.

Why did Lacan see this situation as unresolvable? Because desire and the law are linked. The id and the superego derive their power from one another. If one does not exist, neither does the other. Lacan flipped Nietzsche on his head when Lacan said, if God is dead, nothing is permitted. The object Lacan relates to desire is *Das Ding*, or The Thing. Lacan (1986, p. 83) wrote:

> Is the Law the Thing? Certainly not. Yet I can only know of the Thing by means of the Law. In effect, I would not have had the idea to covet it if the Law hadn't said: "Thou shalt not covet it." But the Thing finds a way by producing in me all kinds of covetousness thanks to the commandment, for without the Law the Thing is dead. But even without the Law, I was once alive. But when the commandment appeared, the Thing flared up, returned once again, I met my death. And for me, the commandment that was supposed to lead to life turned out to lead to death, for the Thing found a way and thanks to the commandment seduced me; through it I came to desire death.

Lacan tricked his audience a bit, because he quoted Romans 7, but replaced the word *sin* with *Thing*. He did so to illustrate this connection between the law and The Thing. When Rahner talked about making a free choice, this choice is dependent on multiple options. If there was no law, there would be no choice, only action. This is why original sin remains today. It no longer has the final say over postmortal existence, but it provides part of the basic structure of our freedom in this life.

If integration of the split parts is impossible, if evolution or progress in consciousness does not resolve the guilt, if behavioral coping strategies do not change the *existenstiells*, if original sin cannot be resolved to achieve harmony, what is left to accomplish? How are people to meet up anew with their desire? Mental health is not about the resolution of this fundamental conflict. As Vergote (1988, p. 26) wrote, "The absence of conflict is not, however, a sign of psychic health. All personal suffering can be avoided by evading troublesome demands, but in doing so one will extinguish the vita force of all personal desire as well." Getting to the truth of desire and resolving it are contradictory goals. The task is to speak about this conflict. One must put this conflict into words.

Lacan was not interested in helping patients become happy. He was not interested in helping them develop self-control or give free reign to their every desire. Lacan did not want to psycho-educate his patients. Lacan wanted his patients to speak and to hear themselves. When patients bring their symptoms, and clinicians conceptualize them as representing unconscious conflict, between what they want and what they ought not to want, between who they are and who they think they ought to be, Lacan (1986, p. 311) provided a foundational question to prompt reflection: "Have you acted in conformity with the desire that is in you?"

Lacan did not advocate everyone act on every desire all the time. The question is designed to probe the unconscious, get people thinking about their actions and their relationship to their desires. There are times when it makes sense to act in conformity with desire, and there are times when, for one reason or another, one should not act in conformity with desire. But there is a question behind this question: what is my unconscious desire? How can anyone know? Lacan saw much of humanity as trying to resolve or repress the conflict rather than confront it, speak about it. The Church led by Pius XII was a clear example. But this approach leads to repetition compulsion. It restricts freedom to make a choice. Instead, Lacan directed us back to all the signs Freud identified: slips of the tongue, bungled actions, dreams, etc.

The command from the primal father to his sons was correlative to a desire. What the sons wanted, more than what their father *possessed,* was to *be* their father. If the reader understands the father to be a God figure, then Adam in Genesis held a similar desire. The Lutheran theologian Dietrich Bonhoeffer (1997, pp. 111–113) described Adam as wanting to become *sicut Deus,* like God.

What does it mean to be God, at least for Adam? To be whole (not to lack), to possess all knowledge, and to be all powerful, that is, without limits. But because God is not human, to become God is to stop being human, in other words, to die.

To desire to *be* God, *sicut deus,* is to reject *imago dei,* the *image* of God in humanity. Desire is therefore a reflection of identification. Adam unconsciously rejected something in himself which he hoped would be eliminated through his acting out in the eating of the fruit. There was a fantasy which preceded the action. Therefore, original sin can only be understood through a recognition of original desire.

Lacan (1986, p. 321) argued guilt, from a psychoanalytic perspective, is intimately related to this desire. Lacan argued, provocatively, that "the only thing of which one can be guilty is of having given ground relative to one's desire." Again, it is not moral or immoral to give ground to one's desire. There are consequences either way. It is a question of how aware people are of giving ground, how they justify it to themselves.

Justification is both a psychoanalytic and theological task. Sins are like symptoms in how they restrict human freedom. This freedom necessarily entails the acceptance of limits. Humans are not deities and must give up the fantasy of omnipotence. If the story of Eden illustrates the birth of consciousness, it also illustrates the birth of the unconscious, and the conflict between them.

People must recognize themselves to be in a position where they must justify their actions considering their desire. For Rahner, that is before God, for Lacan, it is to the unconscious. Rahner saw many Christians in his era attempting to skirt this issue in the attempt to resolve the sense of guilt he saw as ineradicable. Redemption is not the human task. Freedom, on this side of eternity, is not about being entirely resolved of sin or redeemed from it. Freedom is a constant struggle to say yes to the image of God within humanity rather than pursue another image which denies humanity.

Guilt, for Lacan, is when people have given ground relative to their unconscious desire. For Rahner, guilt is the closing of oneself to God's self-communication, or God's desire. Psychoanalysis and a life of faith consist in individuals confronting their desire, in taking account of who they are, what they want, and justifying the actions they take to address the conflicts which inevitably arise between identity and desire. Existing East of Eden, all people must determine how to relate to this psychic split.

References

Boersma, H. (2009). *Nouvelle théologie and sacramental ontology: A return to mystery.* Oxford University Press.

Bonhoeffer, D. (1997). *Creation and fall: A theological exposition of Genesis 1–3*. In John. W. de Gruchy (Ed.), *Dietrich Bonhoeffer Works*, Vol. 3. Fortress Press.

Boyer, C. (1940). Qu'est que la théologie: Réflexions sur une controverse. *Greg*, 21: 255–266.

Bridgman, L. & Carter, J. (1989). Christianity and psychoanalysis: Original sin - oedipal or preoedipal? *Journal of Psychology and Theology*, 17(1): 3–8.

D'Ambrosio, M. (1991). Ressourcement theology, aggiornamento, and the hermeneutics of tradition. *Communio*, 18: 530–553.

Del Colle, R. (2010). Neo-Scholasticism. In D. Ferguson (Ed.), *The Blackwell companion to nineteenth-century theology* (pp. 375–394.). Blackwell Publishing.

Dempsey, P. (1951). The first sin. (M. Choisy, Trans.). *Psyché*, 57–58: 485–496.

Freud, S. (1913). Totem and taboo. In J. Strachey (Ed. & Trans.), *The standard edition of the complete psychological works of Sigmund Freud*, Vol, 13. Hogarth Press.

Kertelge, K. (1991). The sin of Adam in the light of Christ's redemptive act according to Romans 5:12–21. *Communio*, 18: 502–513.

Lacan, J. (1986). *The seminar of Jacques Lacan, Book VII: The ethics of psychoanalysis, 1959–1960*. (J.A. Miller, Ed. & D. Porter, Trans.). Norton.

Lacan, J. (2007). The function and field of speech and language in psychoanalysis. In J. Lacan, *Ecrits: The first complete edition in English* (pp. 197–268). (B. Fink, Trans.). W.W. Norton.

Lacan, J. (2013). *The triumph of religion: Preceded by discourse to Catholics.* (B. Fink, Trans.). Polity Press.

Leo XIII (1879). Aeterni patris [Encyclical letter]. Vatican. https://www.vatican.va/content/leo-xiii/en/encyclicals/documents/hf_l-xiii_enc_04081879_aeterni-patris.html.

Parente, P. (1942, February 9–10). Nouve tendenze teologiche, *L'Osservatore Romano.*

Pius XII (1950). Humani generis [Encyclical letter]. Vatican. https://www.vatican.va/content/pius-xii/en/encyclicals/documents/hf_p-xii_enc_12081950_humani-generis.html.

Rahner, K. (1982). *Foundations of Christian faith: An introduction to the idea of Christianity.* (W. Dych, Trans.). The Crossroad Publishing Company.

Schneider, A. (2024). "Making the holy obscene": A thematic analysis of Freudian psychoanalysis in the Catholic press. *Integratus,* 2(1): 13–36.

Vergote, A. (1988). *Guilt & desire: Religious attitudes and their pathological derivatives.* (M.H. Wood, Trans.). Yale University Press.

Vitz, P. & Gartner, J. (1989). Christianity and psychoanalysis, part 1: Jesus as the anti-oedipus. *Journal of Psychology and Theology,* 12(1): 4–14.

Wiedenhofer, S. (1991). The main forms of contemporary theology of original sin. *Communio,* 18: 514–529.

Chapter 6

"Say the Word and my Soul Shall be Healed"

Ethical Speech in Catholicism and Psychoanalysis

Speech in the Gospel of Matthew

> When he entered Capernaum, a centurion came to him, appealing to him and saying, "Lord, my servant is lying at home paralyzed, in terrible distress." And he said to him, "I will come and cure him." The centurion answered, "Lord, I am not worthy that you should enter under my roof; but only speak the word, and my servant will be healed."
>
> (Matt. 8:5–8)

"Say the word and my soul shall be healed." This line adapted from the Gospel of Matthew is recited during each Liturgy of the Eucharist by the congregation prior to receiving the Eucharist. The theological interpretation of the Roman centurion's story revolves around worthiness, trust, and authority. The centurion evidently believed that Jesus did not need to be physically present to enact the healing of his servant. He recognized Jesus' divine authority and therefore understood he was underneath Jesus in the hierarchy and trusted that Jesus' power would extend wherever Jesus held authority, in this case, his home and his servant.

The centurion felt unworthy to have Jesus in his home. But he still requested action from Jesus. "Say the word," urged the centurion. He identified the effectual mechanism of cure. Jesus did not walk to the centurion's home and touch his servant, as Jesus had done in multiple other cases. Instead, the servant was healed through the speech of Jesus. "And to the centurion, he said, 'Go, let it be done for you according to your faith.' And the servant was healed in that hour" (Matt. 8:13). Jesus' speech healed the servant within an hour.

This story is not the sole case of healing through speech. In the passages which follow this one in Matthew, Jesus "cast out the spirits *with a word*," (Matt 8:16), he "*rebuked* the winds and the sea," (Matt. 8:26), he *said* "Go" and demons came out of the two men and into a herd of swine (Matt. 8:28–34). To the paralytic, Jesus *said*, "Stand up, take your bed and go to your home" (Matt. 9:6). To the man with a withered hand, Jesus *told* him, "Stretch out your hand" (Matt. 12:13). He "*rebuked*" the demon in a boy and the boy was healed "instantly" (Matt. 17:17).

DOI: 10.4324/9781003485346-8

In reverse, the woman who was suffering from hemorrhages *said* out loud, "If only I touch his cloak, I will be made well" (Matt. 9:20) and Jesus indicated it was not her touch, but her faith, that made her well. The Canaanite woman *persuaded* Jesus through her persistent speech to heal her daughter. In many of these stories, Jesus is impressed, amazed, moved with compassion, and delighted by peoples' faith articulated through their speech.

Speech, Jesus told his followers, reveals the state of the heart (Matt. 12:34). It is through speech, "by your words," people will be justified and condemned on the day of judgment (Matt. 12:37). The mechanism of healing and of change more broadly was speech. Jesus his speech from the signs people sought from him. He welcomed the speech but condemned the demand for signs (Matt. 12:39, 16:4).

Jesus asked his disciples, "Who do you *say* that I am?" Jesus did not ask who his disciples *believed* him to be but wanted them to speak about their belief. It was when Peter put his belief into words that Jesus recognized him as the rock on which the Church would be built (Matt. 16:17–20). It was Peter's verbal denial of Jesus which fulfilled Jesus' prophecy and led Peter to weep bitterly (Matt. 26:75).

There are also times when Jesus asked people *not* to speak about him. Jesus instructed the leper he healed to *not* tell anyone (Matt 8:4). In the Gospel of Mark, he commanded the witnesses of his healing of the deaf-mute man to *not* tell anyone (they did so anyway) (Mark 7:36). After the passage when Peter confessed Jesus as Christ, Jesus admonished the disciples not to tell anyone he was the Christ (Matt. 16:20). While the grouping of these passages under the theory of the "Messianic Secret" has been debated in the past, these passages reinforce the power of speech. Jesus knew the power of the spoken title of Christ and how speaking it aloud would change the lives of those who spoke it and heard it.

Time and again, Jesus revealed it is not enough to believe in him, but to speak about him, to him. Later in Matthew, Jesus obviously saw that two men who asked him for mercy were blind, yet he wanted them to voice their desire for healing. Jesus asked the, "What do you want me to do for you?" There are no self-evident needs or meeting of needs in the gospels. One must speak.

The power of speech is also evident in the mass. The Eucharist, the "fount and apex of the whole Christian life" (Levering, 2021, p. 59), is the preeminent example of the power of speech, especially the speech of Christ. As Bishop Robert Barron wrote:

> For Catholic theology, this efficacious word of Christ has not passed out of existence or evanesced into a vague historical memory. Rather, it endures in the Church: in its preaching, its teaching, its sacraments, and above all in the Eucharistic liturgy.
>
> (Vogt, 2020, p. 154)

The speech of Christ was not only a historical event of which there is a written record, but his speech is also a present and future reality through the authority he bestowed on the disciples and those who were ordained after them. As the examples from Matthew make clear, while there is a unique power in the words of Jesus and in the clergy, the speech of laypeople is efficacious too. Why else would they need to speak during mass? From the penitential rite to the recitation of the Creed, through the Lord's prayer and the passing of peace, laypeople's speech makes an impact.

The same is true in the other sacraments. In baptism, the priest speaks "In the name of the Father, Son, and Holy Spirit," and the parents and the congregation speak the renewal of their baptismal vows, and the parents speak their commitments to their child. In confirmation, catechumens profess their faith and renounce sin as they become full members of the Church.

In reconciliation, the penitent verbally confesses their sins and the priest, *in persona Christi,* verbally absolves their sins. In marriage, the couple declares their consent to one another and the priest blesses the rings and the couple. Finally, during the sacrament of Holy Orders, the bishop speaks his consecratory prayer over the candidate for ordination. The elect must "declare before the people" their "intention to undertake this office" (United States Conference of Catholic Bishops, 2021, p. 73). Speech is an essential component of every Catholic sacrament.

None of this focus on speech should detract from the importance of the body in scripture. Jesus inaugurated a fundamentally new relationship to the human body through his incarnation. He also healed and blessed through his touch and taught his disciples to do likewise. He is the embodied Word of God. Human speech is dependent on the mind and body to become articulated.

Michel de Certeau

Michel de Certeau (1925–1986) was a French historian and philosopher who was educated in Grenoble and Lyon. He then was admitted to the seminary in Lyon and joined the Society of Jesus in 1950 and became an ordained priest in 1956. About a decade later, de Certeau was a founding member of the École Freudienne de Paris with psychoanalyst Jacques Lacan in 1964. Though not a trained psychoanalyst, with brief periods of personal analysis, de Certeau nevertheless cited psychoanalytic literature and theory throughout his published works.

Pope Francis described his spiritual and theological development as heavily influenced by French thinkers (Denis, 2016). Perhaps this influence is not surprising, given the origins of the Society of Jesus. But Francis cited men who were alive during his theological studies as most important. "In my theological reflection, I have always been nourished by Henri de Lubac and Michel de Certeau. For me, de Certeau remains the greatest theologian for today" (Denis, 2016).

For Pope Francis to have cited these two theologians together (and, in other texts, Rahner as well) and identified de Certeau as "the greatest" theologian for today, demonstrates the extent to which Francis was influenced by the *nouvelle theologie* group and those who carried forth the insights and interpretations they taught. Their importance for the present, through de Certeau, also reveals that Francis understood the changes this theological movement sought for the Church are still needed today.

For de Certeau, being a Catholic theologian influenced by and actively participating in psychoanalysis was not an easy role. As David Wootton (2001) described in his review of de Certeau's works titled *Lacanian Jesuit*: "To be a Jesuit is difficult; to be a Lacanian is hard work; to be both at once is something extraordinary, for two more demanding collectivities could scarcely be found."

To describe de Certeau as Lacanian is somewhat inaccurate. There are few references to Lacan in de Certeau's texts but plenty of references to Freud. As Lacan once described himself as Freudian, one must consider de Certeau on similar grounds. Yet Lacan provided de Certeau with a contemporary voice and practice which was distinct from Freud in its Catholic background and de Certeau nimbly analogized much of Lacan's theory into Catholic theology.

De Certeau came to articulate the importance of speech following the student-worker revolution in France in May 1968. Up to 500,000 people who participated in the revolution marched throughout Paris and occupied university campuses, public and private work sites, and governmental buildings (Feenberg & Freedman, 2001). At its height, almost a third of the nation's workforce went on strike, crippling the country's transportation network and the economy overall (Feenberg & Freedman, 2001).

Speech, its encouragement or its suppression, was a political and social act. As de Certeau's colleague Giard summarized in his introduction of de Certeau's work: "Speech is what grants entry into the concert of voices where partial, contradictory, or inchoate truths confront, contradict, and complete one another" (De Certeau, 1997, p. xiii). The revolution was later characterized as "symbolic" rather than "political" because there was little change in political governance.

De Certeau (1997, p. 5), however, understood the symbolic nature of the revolution somewhat differently: "A *symbolic* revolution, therefore, either because it *signifies* more than it effectuates, or because of the fact that it contests given social and historical *relations* in order to create authentic ones." Political change is not all the revolution was about. The power once assumed in the government was observed to be tenuous and temporary. Those who felt powerless suddenly felt significant power. All the literal movements taken by the protestors "aimed at an effect of language" (De Certeau, 1997, p. 7).

The subversive nature of their actions was contained in their equal but opposite push against the meaning of unquestioned societal values: patriotism, culture, profit, etc. The government was restored, but without the illusion of power it once held and with this speech decisively entering history. De Certeau (1997, p. 8) concluded the revolution "was a way out of a heretofore ineffable malaise and of a 'repressed voice.'" Repressed voices found a way to become articulated. "From the beginning to the end, speech is what has played the decisive role" in the lifting of malaise and repression, of opening the possibility of new perspectives (De Certeau, 1997, p. 6). Speech is a revolution in that it upsets the calcified narrative of conscious identity.

Though de Certeau did not refer to theology in his analysis of May 1968, there is a parallel to his religion's history and theology. The revolution of May 1968, as with many other revolutions, recalled the revolution prophesized by Israelites thousands of years ago. Following their exile, many Israelites believed the Messiah who was prophesied to arrive in ancient Palestine was going to usher in a political revolution: topple the Roman Empire, restore Israel as a nation, and rule as an earthly King. When Jesus began to teach about himself as the fulfillment of messianic prophecy, his Jewish followers expected him to fulfill their desire for political revolution. After the crucifixion, the disciples on the road to Emmaus lamented, "we had hoped that he was the one to redeem Israel" (Luke 24:21).

As de Certeau (1983, p. 33) wrote:

> The Jewish tradition is rooted in the biological, familial and social reality of a present and identifiable "body" distinguished from others by "election," a body persecuted through endless wanderings, a body transcended by Scriptures marking on it an unknowable sign.

The Jewish anticipation of a political Messiah was responsive to their bodily suffering, their seemingly endless persecutions beginning with their exile, being unable to govern themselves. Their idea of a revolution, then, was rooted in the restoration of what they lost: a nation defined by their biological identity, familial relations, and social laws. De Certeau (1983, p. 33) continued:

> But Christianity received its form of being apart from its ethnic origin, with a break from its heredity. The "separation" giving rise to the Christian Logos has as an index the very loss of the body which should hold the place of all others, that of Jesus, so that the "evangelical" word, born of this disappearance, must itself take charge of the creation of ecclesiastical, doctrinal or "glorious" bodies destined to be substitutes for the absent body. The word itself becomes the source of a "sacrament" in place of the body.

De Certeau made a distinction between the Jewish sign and the Christian Word. The successful revolution brought about by Christ was not concrete, not legal, not political, but ontological, that is, it revolutionized the nature of what it meant to be human. When the Pharisees and Sadducees demanded a sign from Jesus, he told them, "An evil and adulterous generation asks for a sign, but no sign will be given to it except the sign of Jonah" (Matt. 16:4). The sign of Jonah refers, of course, to the prophet Jonah, who was swallowed by a whale when he refused to speak to the Ninevites. In some sense, Jesus seemed to distinguish between the *demand* of the Pharisees and Sadducees from the Other and the *desire* which emerges from the speech of the subject.

The Gospel of John begins with its proclamation that the Word of God became flesh. The incarnation initiated this change in the flesh of Christ, but also, those who believed Jesus was the Word would become children of God, "who were born, not of blood, nor of the will of the flesh, nor of the will of a man, but of God" (John 1:13). That is, children of God did not become so via biological processes, family affiliation, social standing, or religious authority, but through identification with the Word. This identification produced change.

As Eugene Peterson paraphrased in *The Message*, "But whoever did want him, who believed he was who he claimed and would do what he said, He made to be their true selves" (John 1:9–13). The Word would make them their true selves. To be one's true self is, therefore, to be Christlike.

Jesus was not, despite popular secular commentary, a zealot or a politician. He did not seek to change the immediate judicial or executive framework governing society. Yet he called into question many of the social and religious practices of his day. When he spoke to the Samaritan woman at the well (and asked her to speak to him), he transgressed gender and ethnic norms. When he touched a leper, he transgressed Jewish cleanliness law. When he encouraged children to come to him, he transgressed family norms. When he declared himself the Son of God, the Christ, he called into question the political and religious authorities. The speech of the Word made flesh facilitated "the concert of voices where partial, contradictory, or inchoate truths confront, contradict, and complete one another" (de Certeau, 1997, p. xiii) Jesus facilitated the speech of those on the margins. Such speech led to Jesus' arrest, trial, conviction, and death.

The Anglican Bishop N.T. Wright (2016) characterized Christ's crucifixion as "The day the revolution began." The life, teaching, death, and resurrection of Jesus was understood to usher in a fundamentally new way of being. Though Jesus was killed, and the religious and governmental authority continued to hold power after they killed him, his speech could not be removed from history.

The speech of Christ was orally repeated, recorded in manuscripts, and recited through services outlined as early as the Didache. The change initiated by the speech of Christ was permanent. All things came into being through the Word, nothing existed apart from the Word, and the speech of the Word made flesh changed the people who heard it and spoke about it.

De Certeau (1988, p. 137) made clear the Bible as it was produced in the early Christian centuries was considered speech:

> Before the "modern" period, that is, until the sixteenth or seventeenth century, this writing (Holy Scripture) speaks. The sacred text is a voice, it teaches, it is the advent of a "meaning" on the part of a God who expects the reader (in reality, the listener) to have a "desire to hear and understand" on which access to truth demands.

Before the printing press, few people had access to written scripture. They needed to attend church services and hear the scripture proclaimed to them and vocally respond as they were taught to do so. De Certeau argued access to truth was dependent on scripture being spoken and heard.

The relationship to the text changed in the modern era.

> One can no longer hear it. "Truth" no longer depends on the attention of a receiver who assimilates himself to the great identifying message... There is a disappearance of the places established by a spoken word, a loss of the identities that people believed they received from a spoken word. A work of mourning. Henceforth, identity depends on the production, on the endless moving on (or detachment and cutting loose) that this loss makes necessary. Being is measured by doing.
>
> (De Certeau, 1988, p. 137)

Being is measured by doing, not by hearing someone speak what has already been done. While some in the Church wish for a return to the Latin mass, the higher priority is that the gospel be spoken aloud, people attend mass to hear it and then speak in their communities as extensions of Christ. To live the Christian life, much more than doing the right behaviors, is to hear and speak Christ in community with others.

Full and Empty Speech in Lacanian Psychoanalysis

Jacques Lacan staked his unique position in his paper given at the Rome Congress of Romance Language Psychoanalysts. His psychoanalytic *ressourcement* – a break with the psychoanalytic establishment at that time – was a return to the terminology of Freud and an innovation in the distinction between speech and language in psychoanalytic practice. Lacan (2007, p. 206) stated, "Whether it wishes to be an agent of healing, training, or sounding the depths, psychoanalysis has but one medium: the patient's speech."

The reason Lacan made such a bold claim was he saw psychoanalysts, especially in the United States, become more aligned with biological etiologies and strategies of adaptation of the ego. Lacan (2007, p. 201) stated, "One can trace over the years a growing aversion regarding the functions of speech and the field of language." In the U.S., analysis had been "inflected toward the adaptation of the individual to the social environment, the search for behavior patterns, and all the objectification implied in the notion of 'human relations'" (Lacan, 2007, p. 204).

This aversion to speech and language was, for Lacan, a consequence of the attraction of something opposed to speech – images. As Hook and De Kesel (2022, p. 64) conceptualized the opposition in their commentary on Lacan's text:

> What you have taken as central to psychoanalysis (its ostensibly biological underpinnings or the central role of the ego) is misguided inasmuch as it reads and prioritizes a gestalt (the visual impression of a constellation) over the symbolic operations of language and speech which are of far greater importance.

Lacan placed the field of speech and language within his Symbolic register versus the focus on behavior and gestalts which is within the Imaginary register. For Lacanian psychoanalysis, change occurs by working within the Symbolic register.

Why? Personal identity and interpersonal dynamics occur through the medium of the Symbolic. It is through speech and language, its elaboration through law, culture, and family structures, that subjectivity emerges. People understand themselves and relate to others based on the signifiers with which they identify and those they reject. As Johnston (2024) argued, "Individual subjects are what they are in and through the mediation of the socio-linguistic arrangements and constellations of the register of the Symbolic." An important example are family names and terms. As Lacan (2007, pp. 229–230) illustrated:

> Without names for kinship relations, no power can institute order of preferences and taboos that knot and braid the thread of lineage through the generations. And it is the confusion of generations which, in the Bible as in all traditional laws, is cursed as being the abomination of the Word and the desolation of the sinner.

Words define relationships and power dynamics and facilitate the regulation and implementation of laws. De Certeau's distinction between the sign and the Word is relevant here. Signs do not require any truth of the subject to be created and displayed. They are not implicated in them. Speech necessarily reveals something about the subject. For example, Jesus criticized people who presented with the appearance or gestalt of fasting, but this image *concealed* the truth about them (Matt. 6:16).

The demand for a sign from the Pharisees and Sadducees mirrored the Pharaoh's demand for a sign from Moses and Aaron (Exodus 7). In this story, the Pharaoh's priests performed signs like the ones produced by Aaron and

Moses. The rod became a snake for Aaron and Moses and for the Egyptian priests and the Nile became blood, through the power of Yahweh for Moses and through the "secret arts" for the Egyptians. As a result of this tit for tat, the Pharaoh was unconvinced of the truth. Even when the sign of the frogs convinced Pharaoh to release the people of Yahweh, the Pharaoh himself did not change his religion.

Lacan, through his insistence on the importance of the Symbolic register, taught that the psychoanalyst cannot successfully work via a tit for tat situated in the Imaginary register. One reason for this insistence is that any presentation along the Imaginary is not self-evident. Making a conclusion about a presented affect, for example, involves significant assumptions on the part of the analyst.

When someone cries, it is not necessarily indicative of sadness. The only way to begin to probe the meaning of this affect is to encourage the patient to speak about it. Checking the "flat" box on a psychiatric mental status exam of possible affects reveals only the impression the clinician has of his or her reality of the patient; it reveals next to nothing about the truth of the patient's subjectivity. "The subject – contrary to the tenets of behaviorism – needs to be viewed as fundamentally cultural and not simply as a natural or adaptational entity" (Hook & De Kesel, 2022, p. 17). A cultural view necessarily entails language and history, that is, speaking about the past in the present.

As Miller (2011, p. 52) argued, attention to spoken words "involve[s] less of a leap of theoretical faith than does the more common approach which takes as its source the inferred content of the patient's speech and behavior." Speech is the most observable and accessible provision from the patient in session. Fink (2011) illustrated a case example when he reflected a patient's polyvalent speech back to the patient. Fink was clear that "I did not in any way claim that I saw the *reality* of his" speech (2011, p. 4, emphasis added). Objective reality is not the aim of analysis.

According to Lacan (2007, p. 213):

> What is at stake is not reality, but truth, because the effect of full speech is to reorder past contingencies by conferring on them the sense of necessities to come, such as they are constituted by the scant freedom through which the subject makes them present.

The concept of full speech will be elaborated below, but for now it is enough to recognize that reality is a perceptual (i.e. imaginal) experience versus speech which organizes and reorganizes the history of the individual.

For Fink, both analyst and patient were confronted with objective speech which held potentially unconscious material, that is, truth. Fink (2011, p. 4) went on to conclude:

> There is something about the polyvalence of a completed speech act, something about the multiple meanings of formulations as they were

> enunciated in the course of a session, that can be shown to other people as evidence of split or multiple intentionality, as evidence of the split between conscious and unconscious.

Spoken speech produces an objective text which can be repeated, explored, and questioned, in ways that a "lived experience" of momentary emotional connection cannot be done.

Important for this approach is that pointing to the ambiguity of a spoken statement is not typically a relief to the neurotic patient but often disturbs the deeply held beliefs (schemas, imagos) they have constructed about themselves and other people. The spoken Word is a disruptive, not a pacifying, act. Lacan was familiar with the *logos* discourse that begins the Gospel of John. In *Discourse to Catholics*, Lacan (2013, p. 74) wrote:

> I am in favour of John and his "In the beginning was the Word," but it is an enigmatic beginning. It means the following: for the average Joe – for this carnal being, this repugnant personage – the drama begins only when the Word is involved, when it is incarnated, as the true religion says. It is when the Word is incarnated that things really start going badly. Man is no longer at all happy, he no longer resembles at all a little dog who wags his tail or a nice monkey who masturbates. He no longer resembles anything. He is ravaged by the Word.

This statement seems counterintuitive at first glance. Why would Jesus' incarnation, understood by Christians to be the beginning of salvation history, be the moment "things really start going badly?" To help understand Lacan's point, a second question is necessary: for whom did things really start going badly? One easy answer is the religious and political authorities whom Jesus questioned time and time again.

Yet it would be too convenient to locate the drama solely with the powerful leaders. The disruption of the Word affects everyone. When Lacan said that man "no longer resembles anything," what he meant is that Imaginary identifications have broken apart. People are not who they thought or who they said they were. They are not dogs with a wagging tail, obedient to the law. They are not masturbating monkeys, simply behaving on instinct. They no longer resemble, that is, depict, a gestalt. They lack. The Word puts into question the egos that have been constructed, adapted, and defended in the pursuit of illusory wholeness. The Word directs attention to the lack, the source of desire.

Not all speech, however, gets at the truth of the individual. Lacan distinguished between empty and full speech. Full speech is also considered true speech, but truth in this context is not an objective fact. Telling a lie, for example, is not true in the sense of reality, but can be considered full speech if it reveals something of the truth of the individual. As Lacan (2007, p. 209) wrote, "Even if it communicates nothing, discourse represents the existence of communication; even if it denies the obvious, it affirms that speech constitutes truth; even if it is destined to deceive, it relies on faith in testimony." When a patient tells a lie, the content of the lie may contain much more of their subjective truth than they intend. On the other hand, a patient may tell an entirely accurate story without communicating anything of the truth.

One difference between full and empty speech is where the speech leads. "Empty speech has an alienating destination, even if composed of factually true fragments; full speech, by contrast, can be error ridden, may involve falsities and untruths en route to a moment of revelation" (Hook & De Kesel, 2022, p. 71). While plenty of speech is designed to obfuscate truth, speech is nonetheless the vehicle for truth and cannot help but lead to truth if the listener knows when to punctuate the speech and the speaker is willing to engage the ambiguity of their speech.

Discernment (a term which has Catholic and psychoanalytic utility) is necessary for the analyst to distinguish between full and empty speech. Lacan (2007, p. 209) argued:

> The point [of analytic intervention] is to figure out to which "part" of this discourse the significant term is relegated, and this is how [Freud] proceeds in the best of cases: he takes the description of an everyday event as a fable addressed as a word to the wise, a long prosopopoeia as a direct interjection, and, contrariwise, a simple slip of the tongue as a highly complex statement, and even the rest of a silence as the whole lyrical development it stands in for.

Lacan argued, via Freud, that true or full speech means something more than what is consciously intended. But that discourse must be acted upon, brought to the patient's attention, for it to have an impact. "It is, therefore, a propitious punctuation that gives meaning to the subject's discourse" (Lacan, 2007, p. 209). Speech into a void does not produce change. Symbolic mediation is necessary to reach the truth of the unconscious.

What is the unconscious? For Lacan (2007, p. 215), "The unconscious is the chapter of my history that is marked by a blank or occupied by a lie: it is the censored chapter." The unconscious is a censored truth. This phenomenon is contrary to how censorship has been utilized in the Catholic Church. The Index of Forbidden Books, discussed in chapter four, was a method for censoring words the Church believed to be false, including psychoanalytic theory.

Yet Freud taught that repression is always only partially successful. As Lacan (2007, p. 215) put it: "But the truth can be refound; most often it has already been written elsewhere. Namely, in monuments (body), in archival documents (childhood memories), in semantic evolution (my vocabulary), in traditions (conveyance of history), and in its traces (exegesis)." One's personal history and body cannot be completely censored. People must relate to their history in some way.

> What we teach the subject to recognize as his unconscious is his history – in other words, we help him complete the current historicization of the facts that have already determined a certain number of the historical 'turning points' in his existence.
>
> (Lacan, 2007, p. 217)

How people go about forgetting their history (through repression, projection, substitution, etc.) contributes to the trajectory, form, and content of their psychic structures. "It is not a question of biological memory, nor of its intuitionist mystification, nor of the paramnesia of the symptom, but of remembering, that is, of history" (Lacan, 2007, p. 213). In the construction of the ego, parts of peoples' histories are left out to create the illusion of wholeness called the self. Despite the popular psychology literature which aims at self-awareness, "The unconscious is that part of concrete discourse qua transindividual, which is not at the subject's disposal in reestablishing the continuity of his conscious discourse" (Lacan, 2007, p. 214). The unconscious is not at one's disposal, that is, it opposes – through symptoms – conscious efforts to control the narrative of one's lives.

While the ego is the "self-serving" narrative left over after the unconscious has been edited, "what constitutes me as a subject is my question" (Lacan, 2007, p. 247). What constitutes the subject is not a behavior, not a feeling, and not just any speech, but a question. Indeed, voicing this question, taking the form of a demand of/for the analyst, marks the end of the preliminary sessions and begins the analytic discourse proper (for more detail on preliminary sessions in Freud and Lacan, see Quinet, 1999).

Symptoms, the interruptions in the carefully constructed stories about the ego, are reflective of truths that have yet to be spoken. Those truths must be spoken for the symptoms to resolve. "If Symptoms can be entirely resolved in an analysis of language because a symptom is itself structured like a language: a symptom is language from which speech must be delivered" (Lacan, 2007, p. 223). Not only is the unconscious structured like a language, but so are its symptoms. "A symptom here is the signifier of a signified that has been repressed from the subject's consciousness" (Lacan, 2007, p. 232).

The analyst must listen, but also discern, which signifiers are most important to punctuate. The analyst must use their ears, "which is, according to both physiology and the Gospels, the normal use made of them: having ears in order not to hear, in other words, in order to detect what is to be understood" (Lacan, 2007, p. 211). Lacan here played with a common phrase in Christian scripture. "He who has ears to hear, let him hear" is a phrase spoken by Jesus multiple times in the synoptic gospels of Matthew (11:15; 13:9, 43), Mark (4:9, 23), and Luke (8:8, 14:35). The phrase is also used in the narration of the revelation of Jesus in Revelation (2:7, 11, 17, 29; 3:6, 13, 22; 13:9).

Both Jesus and Lacan seemed aware that ears are not often hearing what is true. As much as there is an emphasis on true speech, there is also a need for true listening. Lacan (2007, p. 211) went on: "For [the analyst] has no other ears, no third or fourth ear designed for what some have tried to describe as a direct transaudition of the unconscious by the unconscious." Lacan here criticized the psychoanalyst Theodor Reik, who authored the book *Listening with the Third Ear* (1948), in which Reik argued psychoanalysts should return, not to Freud's teaching as Lacan sought, but to Freud's self-analysis and self-listening to understand the patient's position through the analyst's unconscious, bypassing the need for speech. Lacan was clear: the focus must be on facilitating the patient's true speech and this must occur with an Other.

In the *Ephphatha* Rite in the liturgy for baptism, priests repeat the actions of Jesus with the deaf man who could barely talk in Mark 7:31–37. Jesus put his fingers in the man's ears, then spits and touches the man's tongue. Priests, in touching the ears and lips of (while not spitting on) their parishioners, indicate there has been a spiritual block against hearing and speaking and so clear the ears and mouth.

Psychoanalysts, without touching or spitting, recognize a similar psychic block and precisely punctuate the words that are being spoken to open the ears of the patient to hear them. "Analysis," Lacan (2007, p. 241) thought, "consists in playing on the multiple staves of the score that speech constitutes in the registers of language." Speech is like a musical score in which multiple levels are being simultaneously performed. Listening to only one level, conscious intention, is akin to being deaf to the unconscious.

Key to this idea is that the unconscious is already being spoken, in part, by the patient. Psychoanalysis does not compose a new score. What patients need help with is listening to themselves.

> In order to free the subject's speech, we introduce him to the language of his desire, that is, to the primary language in which – beyond what he tells us of himself – he is already speaking to us unbeknown to himself.
>
> (Lacan, 2007, p. 243)

Returning to de Certeau (1988, p. 137), Lacan in a sense argued truth depends "on the attention of a receiver who assimilates himself to the great identifying message," in this case, their own spoken signifiers.

Speech, from the patient and the analyst, is not intended "to inform but to evoke" (Lacan, 2007, p. 247). Speech is not, within the psychoanalytic frame, a transmission of information from one speaker to another. Such language is akin to an email. Speech which evokes is speech which brings history into the present. This historization is sought not for the sake of understanding the past but to clarify one's desire for the future. As Lacan (2007, p. 249) said, "Analysis can have as its goal only the advent of true speech and the subject's realization of his history in is relation to a future." Choosing when to end the session is therefore "a punctuation of [the patient's] progress" towards the clarification of their unconscious desire.

Catholic Versus Psychoanalytic Speech

With speech being of central importance for both Catholicism and psychoanalysis, scholars have questioned the comparability of their practices (Schneider, 2024). As Oraison (1958, p. 363) noted, "psychoanalysis has gained a considerably wider acceptance in Protestant countries where confession does not exist, than in Catholic countries where it does." The Catholic Church has long recognized the importance of speaking one's sins in the sacrament of reconciliation so the priest *in persona Christi* can hear them, forgive them, and absolve them. Whether psychoanalysis is simply the psychological equivalent of confession, or confession the spiritual equivalent of psychoanalysis, has been a contentious debate.

Contributing to this debate is a confusion of terms. As an example, Father O'Brien (1948, p. 9) argued in his book *Psychiatry and Confession*, "Psychoanalysis had its origin in the discovery of the therapeutic effects of confessing or revealing the secret causes of inner discords to a sympathetic auditor or father confessor." O'Brien essentially conflated not only what is understood to occur via the patient's speech in analysis, but also the role of analyst and priest! O'Brien then concluded that confession is the "best catharsis" (1948, p. 19). If confession and analysis are essentially the same practice, Catholics are not in need of psychoanalysis, nor are non-Catholics in need of confession. If these practices are different, does one conflict or condone the other?

Carl Jung, the analytical psychologist whom Freud had hoped would carry forth his theory after his death, saw no difference between the two practices. Jung stated, "Catholics stand the least in need of the services of a psychoanalyst" because "the Catholic can unload his mental burdens in the confessional" ("Psychoanalyst finds that Catholic needs met by the confessional," 1925, p. 1). Jung focused on the cathartic dimension of psychoanalytic speech. Yet Freud (1964, p. 188) offered a subtle but clear distinction: "In confession the sinner tells what he knows; in analysis the neurotic has to tell more."

The focus on catharsis, sublimation, and confession bypasses the unconscious, what the neurotic sinner does not know. This focus also misses the element of mysticism in theology, that which clergy and laypeople cannot know. A more fruitful comparison, which considers both the unconscious and mystery, is between psychoanalysis and spiritual direction. Murphy (2018) located Lacan's sole reference to spiritual direction in Lacan's essay "Psychoanalysis and its Teaching":

> [T]he perplexities of Spiritual Direction which have been elaborated over the centuries along the path of a demand for truth – a demand linked to no doubt a cruel personification of this Other, but which did a fairly good job of sounding the folds in striving to clear out every other affection from people's loins and hearts.
>
> (Lacan, 2007, p. 381)

The demand for truth Lacan situated in spiritual direction was associated with premodern or ancient Christians. As Murphy (2018, p. 65) argued, "the language of the early Spiritual Directors was marked by an austere linguistic economy. They were rooted in an oral tradition that valued the concise, the immediate, and the provocative." The desert father and mothers practiced speech that did not inform but evoked – called forth – something of God in pilgrims who sought their guidance.

This guidance, the desire for a word, reflects what Lacan would understand as a resolution to alienation. As de Certeau (1983, p. 33) argued:

> In Lacan's circle, the "monk" (monos) and the ascetic of the speech which he upholds (with humor, even with a ferocious irony found in monastic speech patterns), the founder of a "congregation" in a desert labeled as "worldly," all gather together the practitioners of a desire whose truth can liberate those alienated from their identity.

Spiritual directors, then, are attentive to their directees' descriptions of their daily lives and listen for occurrences of God at work in their otherwise alienated experiences of identity. If God and the unconscious are held analogously, then psychoanalysis and spiritual direction have much in common. Within the Ignatian spiritual hour, the Christian is advised, "Be faithful to the hour and its structure and if you are lucky you will encounter God and all hell will break loose!" (Marsh, 2009, p. 36). The irony of hell aside, Christian mystics understood, as Lacan did, that the Word is disruptive. This disruption of the ego's Imaginary identification in the face of mystery allows the individual's desire to be spoken.

In the fifth step of Ignatian prayer, "I ask for what I desire," and "fundamentally *id quod volo*, that which I want, must be honest and arise from real desire" (Marsh, 2009, pp. 34–35). By "real desire" Marsh is not intending a reference to Lacan's register of the Real, but it is a helpful point of intersection. It is the Real which disrupts, which cannot be symbolized, the gap or lack in what people have Symbolized. God is much more associated with the Real than with the Imaginary or Symbolic registers. The name-of-the-father may be Symbolic, but the Father is Real.

Murphy (2023) bridged these two practices, spiritual direction and Lacanian psychoanalysis, with the term "apophatic listening." This listening is aimed at answering the question of the patient's desire.

> What is the answer to [an individual's] Desire lies not in some knowledge of the Abba. Nor does it lie within some internal emotional object. Rather it lies in the fragmented connection between their intentions, thoughts, sense of self, and its relationship to an untameable, excessive Grace.
>
> (Murphy, 2018, p. 66)

Knowledge and affect cannot lead to desire because they serve to repress desire. The Grace of God is Real in that it often does not make sense; it often flies in the face of societal (Symbolic) norms and constructed (Imaginary) identities.

Speech, therefore, in both spiritual direction and psychoanalysis, is not only a political and social act but an ethical act as well. As de Certeau (1983, p. 34) argued, "Ethics is the form of a belief removed from the alienating imagination where it would guarantee the real and shed into speech that which is said by the desire instituted by this lack." Too strict a focus on confession and behavior risks an Imaginary moralism that contributes to repression and suffering.

Though people cannot fully know themselves nor can they say everything, the ethical imperative is to try. As the contemporary philosopher Peter Rollins (2006, p. xii) put it, "When it comes to talking about God, that which we cannot speak of is the one thing about whom and to whom we must never stop talking." The same holds true for talking about the unconscious.

References

De Certeau, M. (1983). Lacan: An ethics of speech. *Representations*, 3: 21–39.

De Certeau, M. (1988). *The practice of everyday life.* (S. Rendell, Trans.). University of California Press.

De Certeau, M. (1997). *The capture of speech & other political writings.* (T. Conley, Trans.). University of Minnesota Press.

Denis, J-P. (2016). Conversation politique avec le pape Francois. *La Vie*. https://www.lavie.fr/christianisme/eglise/conversation-politique-avec-le-pape-franccedilois-13714.php.

Feenberg, A. & Freedman, J. (2001). *When poetry ruled the streets: The French May events of 1968*. State University of New York Press.

Fink, B. (2011). What's so different about Lacan's approach to psychoanalysis? *Psychoanalytic Review*, 98(6): 843–869.

Freud, S. (1964). The question of lay analysis. In J. Strachey (Ed. & Trans.), *The standard edition of the complete psychological works of Sigmund Freud*, Vol. 20 (pp.179–258). Hogarth Press.

Hook, D. & De Kesel, M. (2022). The function and field of speech and language in psychoanalysis. In D. Hook, C. Neill, & S. Vanheule (Eds.), *Reading Lacan's Écrits: From 'Logical Time' to 'Response to Jean Hyppolite'*. Kindle Edition.

Johnston, A. (2024). Jacques Lacan. In E.N. Zalta & U. Nodelman (Eds.), *The Stanford encyclopedia of philosophy.* https://plato.stanford.edu/archives/sum2024/entries/lacan.

Lacan, J. (2007). *Écrits: The first complete edition in English.* (B. Fink, Trans.). W.W. Norton Company.

Lacan, J. (2013). *The triumph of religion preceded by discourse to Catholics.* (B. Fink, Trans.). Polity. (Original work published 2005).

Levering, M. (2021). *The word on fire Vatican II collection,*Vol. 1. Word on Fire Institute.

Marsh, R.R. (2009). Imagining Ignatian spiritual direction. *The Way,* 48(3): 27–42.

Miller, M. (2011). *Lacanian psychotherapy: Theory and practical applications.* Routledge.

Murphy, M. (2018). Dialogue between the clinical practice of Lacanian psychoanalysis and the discipline of spiritual direction. *Vinayasādhana: Dharmaram Journal of Psycho-Spiritual Formation,* 9(1): 58–74.

Murphy, M. (2023). The return to the mystical: Jacques Lacan, John of the Cross, and the Christian tradition. *Church Life Journal.* https://churchlifejournal.nd.edu/articles/the-return-to-the-mystical-jacques-lacan-john-of-the-cross-and-the-christian-tradition/.

O'Brien, J.A. (1948). *Psychiatry and confession: Light on the talking cure of psychoanalysis.* The Paulist Press.

Oraison, M. (1958). The psychoanalyst and the confessor. *CrossCurrents,* 8(4): 363–376.

Psychoanalyst finds that Catholic needs met by the confessional. (1925, January 29). *The Catholic Telegraph.* Retrieved from The Catholic News Archive.

Quinet, A. (1999). The functions of the preliminary interviews. *European Journal of Psychoanalysis,* 8–9.

Reik, T. (1948). *Listening with the third ear; the inner experience of a psychoanalyst.* Farrar, Straus & Co.

Rollins, P. (2006). *How (not) to speak of God.* Paraclete Press.

Schneider, A. (2024). "Making the holy obscene": A thematic analysis of Freudian psychoanalysis in the Catholic Press. *Integratus,* 2(1): 13–36.

United States Conference of Catholic Bishops. (2021). *Ordination of a bishop, of priests, and of deacons.* United States Conference of Catholic Bishops.

Vogt, B. (2020). *The word on fire Bible: the gospels.* Word on Fire.

Wootton, D. (2001). Lacanian Jesuit. *London Review of Books,* 23(19): 31–32.

Wright, N.T. (2016). *The day the revolution began: Reconsidering the meaning of Jesus's crucifixion.* HarperOne.

Part 3

Contemporary Applications

Chapter 7

Rites of Truth

Priestly and Psychoanalytic Formation

The number of priests in the United States is in steady decline (United States Conference of Catholic Bishops (USCCB), 2022, p. 10). Why? Novotny (2023, p. 106) argued, "The double crisis in the Catholic Church caused by instances of sexual abuse and their cover-up by the Church hierarchy calls into question the initial formation of priests and, in particular, the milieu of Catholic seminaries." Therefore, it is prudent to explore the requirements and process for priesthood to determine what aspects hinder or facilitate that formation. This chapter compares the training of Catholic priests in the United States to the training of Lacanian psychoanalysts. The processes are interrogated through primary texts including the *Program for Priestly Formation* (Hereafter *PPF*) (USCCB, 2022) and Jacques Lacan's essays regarding training within and extant to the *Ecríts.*

Historically, psychoanalytic training institutes have struggled to determine how best to form their candidates. Lacan (2007, p. 382) argued "none of the 'institutes' currently sponsored by [psychoanalysis] around the world has yet even tried to put together the curriculum of studies whose intention and extension Freud so often and in such detail defined as allowing for no substitute." The Lacanian tradition has always considered training to be an integral part of its theory. However, as a result of historical conflict and institutional splitting, institutes do not adhere to a uniform application of training (Tardits, 2018). What these various institutes share, however, is that it is not a learned body of knowledge but the process of psychoanalysis itself which produces psychoanalysts.

Candidates for both schools recognize there is something that they do not know about themselves and believe formation will help them encounter that truth. However, whereas seminarians are presupposed to be psychologically healthy, analysands enter formation with symptoms. Seminarians are searching for truth about their calling and its potential unfolding in their lives. Analysands need to interrogate and articulate their unconscious desires. Completed formation does not necessarily lead to priest and analyst but a resolution about that calling and desire.

DOI: 10.4324/9781003485346-10

Application and Admission to Seminary

The *PPF*, the document guiding seminaries in the United States, explicitly detailed the traits required of men acceptable for formation. The applicant must first "give witness" to a "conviction" that God wants them to discern whether they are "really called to the priesthood" (USCCB, 2022, p. 36).

Following a review of sacramental records, an autobiography, a review of psychological and medical assessments, interviews with the man and his family, academic transcripts, background checks, and immigration status, those who make the decision for admission (bishops, major superiors, and rectors) must have "moral conviction" about the health of the applicant. The applicant must possess "overall personal balance, good moral character, a love for the truth, and proper motivation" (USCCB, 2022, p. 35).

Sexuality and gender are subject to "strict vigilance" in this process (USCCB, 2022, p. 33). Only biological men are admitted into seminary formation. Screening is required to determine biological maleness. The candidate must not have "deep seated" homosexuality. Homosexual "tendencies" are not disqualifying but must have been overcome at least three years before ordination to the diaconate (USCCB, 2022, p. 39).

As Berg (2018, p. 13) wrote, "If you're twenty-one and experiencing same-sex attraction, you suffer lots of emotional turbulence. It would be imprudent to allow a man to approach seminary formation with all that turmoil going on inside." Recent literature demonstrates male seminarians think of masculinity in strict biological terms and develop an "essential male inclusivity" to resolve any underlying concerns about their gender (Barnes, 2022).

Applicants should also have no psychopathology, must possess empathy, and have a capacity for friendships and personal growth. The use of psychological testing in applications aims at detecting psychological defects prior to admission. If psychotherapy is recommended, it must be completed prior to admittance or, if needed during formation, the candidate must pause his seminary formation while psychotherapy takes place (USCCB, 2022, p. 43). All internet and social media use are evaluated.

The applicant must not have "committed voluntary homicide," "positively cooperated in a completed abortion," "gravely and maliciously mutilated himself or another," or "attempted suicide" (USCCB, 2022, p. 43). The applicant must not be allergic to wheat and able to consume wine. If the applicant has ever experienced sexual abuse, Church authorities must determine, "with compassionate solicitude for the good of the man and for the good of the Church…whether it is prudent to admit the applicant into a formation program" (USCCB, 2022, p. 44).

Priestly formation presupposes a healthy man. "Indeed, he is called above all to a basic human and spiritual serenity that, by overcoming every form of self-promotion or emotional dependency, allows him to be a man of communion, of mission and of dialogue" (Novotny, 2023, p. 111). As early as his middle to late twenties, this man must have psychological, sexual, and spiritual maturity far beyond his secular peers.

Admission to seminary is therefore predicated on mysterious contradictions: the candidate must be at once intellectually capable but in need of knowledge; sexually mature but committed to renunciation; convinced of his calling but in need of further discernment; psychologically healthy but vigilant for any pathology; a humble sinner in need of grace but without a history of significant harm (as perpetrator or victim).

The new initial stage for priestly formation is the propaedeutic (preliminary) stage. This stage is meant to bridge the gap between the secular world of society and the culture of the Catholic church and its clergy. "Men entering seminary first live in a community separate from the rest of the seminary, do minimal or no coursework, and focus on their human formation and relationship with God" (Dulle, 2024, p. 20).

The candidates withdraw from society and immerse themselves in community, doctrine, scripture, and spiritual practices, what Cullinan (2019, p. 415) called "a basic map of the faith." Individual and group psychotherapy and spiritual direction are available, access to technology is limited and structured, and the men perform work typical of life in a monastery.

This stage aims to develop in the seminarian an "appropriate docility to formation" (USCCB, 2022, p. 57). Humility is only possible when the self that is to be humbled is known well by the individual. As such, "Self-knowledge and awareness are key themes in the area of human formation during the propaedeutic stage" (USCCB, 2022, p. 84). Seminarians must have a sense that they do not know everything about themselves and other people possess the wisdom and direction they need.

To advance past this stage, the seminarian must make "a firm resolution to dedicate himself to the work of priestly formation or, alternatively, to follow a different path in life as a faithful lay Catholic" (USCCB, 2022, p. 58). Having spent a year or more apart from family and friends, studying scripture, engaged in daily prayer and other spiritual practices, the individual is expected to have discerned which path in life to follow.

Admission in Psychoanalytic Formation

The candidate for priestly formation must possess a love for the truth. Anna Freud would have appreciated that standard. In a letter to an aspiring psychoanalyst, she wrote:

> If you want to be a real psychoanalyst you have to have a great love of the truth, scientific truth as well as personal truth, and you have to place this appreciation of truth higher than any discomfort at meeting unpleasant facts, whether they belong to the world outside or to your own inner person.
> (Kohut, 1968, p. 553)

This love of the truth, and its relation to suitability for psychoanalytic formation, proved difficult to qualify and institutionalize. The question of who was qualified to train as a psychoanalyst was contested from the beginning of the profession.

Sigmund Freud (1964b) wrote *The Question of Lay Analysis* to argue against the need for medical training prior to training or practicing as a psychoanalyst. As Tardits (2018, p. 50) argued, what Freud attempted was "to show that the most appropriate training for an analyst is determined by the aims and specific practice of the treatment, which are themselves determined by analytic theory." Psychoanalytic formation is part and parcel of psychoanalytic treatment and theory. Each part informs the other.

While Freud argued a medical education was not a prerequisite to psychoanalytic formation, the qualities of the candidates were not immaterial. As Lacan (1949, p. 430) would later observe, "There is no more difficult task, nor one that deserves more care, than that assumed by the Commission in the selection of candidates for entry." Not everyone who demands formation is provided with it. As Mathew and Hopkins (2023, p. 227) argued, "The important consideration – for many – is the gathering of human experience (one's own, and the learning gleaned from the experience of others), before one is fully qualified to practice."

However, the selection of candidates for entry into the psychoanalytic school was not based on the relative health of the individual. As Sachs (1947, p. 158) argued, "To insist emphatically on such demands as intelligence, honesty, reliability, sufficient professional and cultural training…seems to me unnecessary" because these characteristics apply to any profession. What, if anything, is *unique* about the qualities required of a psychoanalyst? For Sachs (1947, p. 159), the aspiring analyst must possess "the faculty of access to and the will to face his own unconscious." This is both a prerequisite to and a development during one's analysis.

This is not to say that psychoanalysts and institutes have not historically required a range of criteria. During Lacan's work in France, disqualifying factors included intellectual impairment, latent psychosis, mental decompensation, and medical disorders such as epilepsy. Also included were aesthetic abnormalities such as "shocking deformities, visible mutilations or manifest dysfunctions" out of concern for how such images would disrupt the "imaginary support" of the analyst in the transference (Lacan, 1949, p. 430).

Despite Freud's insistence that homosexuality was not morally wrong and belief that people who were homosexual could train as psychoanalysts, institutes, especially in the United States, discriminated against them (Friedman & Downey, 1998; Magee & Miller, 1998; Lewes et al., 2008; Drescher, 2008). Thankfully the heterosexual criterion has been abandoned, with no detriment to the profession.

Lacan oriented the qualifications of an analyst around *the impact on potential analysands* rather than there being an inherent or independent kind of person who is suitable to be an analyst. Training, then, was structured by the dimensions of subjectivity experienced in treatment (Imaginary, Symbolic, Real).

The characteristics which might make someone unsuitable for psychoanalytic training were therefore something to be addressed during the training. "There are always impasses, irresolvable contradictions about the formation of the analyst, and it is impossible to define who can be and what the requirements are to be a 'true' analyst" (Rodríguez, 2019, p. 12). These conflicts are expected, welcomed, and confronted during formation.

The start of personal analysis is the beginning of formation as a psychoanalyst. "The conviction of the rightness of the theory is only acquired in the crucible of one's own analysis, in one's own body and soul" (Tardits, 2018, p. 39). As Freud argued, studying the literature of psychoanalysis is not enough: "They must learn to understand analysis in *the only way that is possible* – by themselves undergoing an analysis" (1964b, p. 248, emphasis added). This requirement remains one of the distinguishing features of psychoanalytic training.

Therefore, the question of criteria for entering formation as a psychoanalyst is to question the criteria for entering psychoanalysis. After Freud, many psychoanalysts focused on who was suitable for psychoanalytic treatment. All the descriptions, according to Miller (2003), oriented around the strength of the ego. Weak or fragile or dependent egos were contraindicated for psychoanalysis. Alternatively, for Lacanians, the sole criterion for admission to psychoanalysis is the "analytical symptom, and a suffering of the symptom" (Miller, 2003, p. 5).

Freud (1964a) identified a preliminary treatment in psychoanalysis which occurred prior to psychoanalysis proper. Freud allotted a few sessions to this endeavor of orientation and clarification before beginning analysis proper. Lacan expanded the preliminary treatment into his notion of preliminary sessions. As Quinet (1999) described, "The expression indicates that there is a threshold, an entry into analysis that is not the same thing as the entrance giving onto the analyst's office."

Fink (1997, p. 13) argued there are multiple tasks during this period. First, the analyst must determine a preliminary diagnosis to determine what direction to take in the treatment. Second, the initial demand must be clarified into an "isolable symptom." A symptom is not a simple complaint or something the analysand wants to remove but a desire to question their current way of understanding themselves and the development of their identity. Preliminary sessions function akin to the propaedeutic stage. The candidate must ask themselves, do they really want to do this work?

Formation in Seminary

The *PPF* detailed four dimensions of priestly formation: human, spiritual, intellectual, and pastoral (USCCB, 2022). There are also stages of formation: propaedeutic, discipleship, configuration, and vocational-synthesis. Each stage of formation is assessed by the growth in the four dimensions.

The *PPF* characterized the goal of the human dimension is for "the human personality of the priest…to be a bridge and not an obstacle" to meeting the needs of the community and "the humanity of the priest is instrumental in mediating the redemptive gifts of Christ to people today" (USCCB, 2022, p. 77). The human dimension is therefore conceptualized in terms of the capacity for selfless relationships.

The human dimension presupposes a capacity for an individual to develop "prudent self mastery" of his sexuality and "renounce" anything which threatens his chastity (USCCB, 2022, p. 81). Spiritual practices are taught to help the seminarian sustain his chastity. Chastity enables the future priest to maintain a posture of charity to his parish and community.

Moral character is another component of the human dimension. The man must be "capable of conversion" (USCCB, 2022, p. 78). Here the *PPF* incorporated psychological theory regarding personality development into its facilitation of the human dimension of priestly development. As Selvam (2019) argued, the *PPF* and other Church documents on priestly formation endorse a "dynamic" understanding of personality. But this dynamic, as stated above, is not a change from pathology to health, but from health to holiness.

The *PPF* reminded formators that:

> formation programs will not be effective for those who manifest extreme inflexibility, narcissism, antisocial behavior or any serious personality disorders or pathology, a lack of sexual integration, deep and unresolved anger (especially against authority), a deep attachment to a materialist lifestyle, or compulsive behaviors or addictions.
>
> (USCCB, 2022, p. 262)

One compelling component of the human dimension should be deeply appreciated by psychoanalysts. "Seminarians bear the primary responsibility for their human formation. The role of the seminary is to assist them in achieving the integral human maturity" (USCCB, 2022, p. 89). The candidate seeks admission to the seminary and needs to know how they intend to make use of it for his formation.

The spiritual dimension is the second dimension in priestly formation. This dimension includes all spiritual practices and the liturgy of the mass. As the *PPF* described, "Spiritual formation is first and foremost a participation in public worship of the Church that is itself a participation in the heavenly Liturgy offered by Christ" (USCCB, 2022, p. 97). There is a need to form in the seminarian a sense of his place in the spiritual landscape. He needs to develop a habit of prayer including private/individual, praying the Liturgy of the Hours with peers, and devotional prayer.

The seminarian's spiritual development involves the "personalized sense of how God's salvation has taken hold of their lives" and how their personal experience fits into the larger Church (USCCB, 2022, p. 99). Participation in the sacraments is an essential element of this process, particularly reconciliation. Unafraid to face his own spiritual struggles, the future priest can put himself at the service of others' spiritual needs. "The seminarian is invited to put everything he is and everything he has at the service of the Gospel, deepening his total self-gift through simplicity of life, celibacy and obedience" (USCCB, 2022, p. 97). The seminarian experiences a shift, or an essential connection, between their personal faith and their responsibility for service.

Biweekly participation in spiritual direction provides ongoing opportunities to reflect and assess their progress. Retreats and other communal activities allow for the time and space to devote themselves to developing these practices. These experiences also develop the interdependence necessary for a well-functioning clergy. Through these activities, the seminarian develops a "simplicity of life" in which he "exercise[s] responsible stewardship over God's creation by using material goods in a way that is both responsive to the call of the Gospel and ecologically responsible" (USCCB, 2022, p. 101). The *PPF* argued that seminarians' spiritual formation is unique in the way in which these men "interiorize the sentiments and ways of acting of Jesus Christ" (USCCB, 2022, p. 97).

Intellectual formation, the third dimension, is not simply the acquisition of academic knowledge about Church history, theology, and ecclesial dynamics. Intellect is here understood as an extension of the mystagogy new Catholics experience in the period after confirmation. This is a knowledge of religious mystery, beginning with Jesus Christ in the Eucharist. Intellectual formation is an empirical determination that what the Church teaches about the Christian mysteries is true in personal experience.

Seminary intellectual formation does not neglect the typical academic curriculum. Seminaries should offer foundational education in the liberal arts which include mathematics, science (natural and human), psychology, history, literature, foreign languages, communication, and fine arts. In addition, training in philosophy and theology with the Catechism as a key text is required. Future priests are expected to learn how to communicate their understanding of theology to their future parishioners and non-Catholics.

Intellectual formation also includes the training in how to pastor. "Seminarians are to learn how to address concerns brought to them by parishioners for whom they can reasonably offer counsel and how to make appropriate referrals for issues beyond their competence" (USCCB, 2022, p. 139). Thus, while priestly formation requires the understanding of what the vocation entails, intellectual formation includes the development of insight into the limits of what a priest can understand and do for their flock. The priest is not all things to all people.

Finally, there is the pastoral dimension of priestly formation. This dimension "requires men who are not self-centered, aloof, judgmental, or self-imposing but instead are characterized by a 'serene openness' and capable of listening and collaboration" (USCCB, 2022, p. 144). There are multiple practical duties the future priest must understand and learn to effectively perform. Preaching, administration of the sacraments, leadership in the parish institution, collaboration with colleagues within and outside of the Church, and community engagement. With so many responsibilities on the horizon, the future priest must develop a tension between their sacrifice/service and their authority to lead.

The seminarian is not thrown into the mix from the outset but engages in a gradual process of greater involvement and responsibility in the sacramental economy. "The seminarian first enters the scene as an observer, then raises questions to understand what is happening, and finally relates it to his other formation" (USCCB, 2022, p. 149). The pastoral dimension requires respect for and understanding of diversity across all aspects of life including religion, culture, politics, age, etc. To that end, future priests must have competency in ministering to people from all walks of life. Pastoral training experiences such as field placements and internships are provided so seminarians have experience with these varied lives.

In addition to the dimensions, there are also stages through which the seminarian moves towards ordination. The propaedeutic stage was described above. That is followed by the discipleship stage, configuration stage, vocational-synthesis stage, and formation ends with ordination in holy orders. What is relevant about these stages for this conversation with psychoanalysis is the mechanism for progression through the stages. The stages are detailed in the *PPF.*

After no less than two years in the discipleship stage, "the seminarian will determine with firm resolve whether God is calling him to present himself for the priesthood" (USCCB, 2022, p. 62). The seminarian receives "positive confirmation" from his formators and is allowed to enter the configuration stage. During the configuration stage, the seminarian develops "greater awareness and personal assumption of priestly identity" (USCCB, 2022, p. 62). The seminarian formally takes on the roles of lector and acolyte. Such a transition means that the candidate has achieved a recognizable mastery over his mind, body, and soul that he can be responsible within a parish setting. After the completion of the configuration stage, the candidate moves out of the seminary and into fulltime parish life.

If at any point during these stages the candidate is not approved to move into the next one, the candidate is "advised to leave the seminary" (USCCB, 2022, p. 76). The *PPF* does not elaborate on why separation from the seminary is advisable in these cases. However, it uses the language of "probation" to refer to this period in which the candidate is given specific goals and the resources necessary to achieve those goals (USCCB, 2022, p. 76). The *PPF* does not provide any examples nor does it describe how a candidate, once in probation, is to be reintegrated into the life of the seminary.

Formation in Psychoanalysis

Freud (1964b, p. 228) provided an outline into how he saw the early formation of psychoanalysts.

> At these institutes the candidates themselves are taken into analysis, receive theoretical instruction by lectures on all the subjects that are important for them, and enjoy the supervision of older and more experienced analysts when they are allowed to make their first trials with comparatively slight cases.

There is no equivalence in psychoanalytic training to the dimensions described above in priestly formation. However, the following dimensions are created for the sake of comparison. Analytic formation includes the ignorance dimension, the linguistic dimension, the technical dimension, and the dimension of desire.

Lacan was critical of the predominant psychoanalytic training model of his day. While he was not the only one concerned about the state of training, he distinguished himself in his critique. Lacan (2007, p. 295) said:

> What is desirable is not that the analysands be more "introspective" but rather that they understand what they are doing; and the remedy is not that the institutes be less structured, but rather that analysts stop dispensing predigested knowledge in them.

This is the ignorance dimension.

Lacan saw training institutes which encouraged candidates to identify with their analysts' egos (to become an analyst like them) and articulate the knowledge of theory that had been, predigested, fed to them. The problem, for Lacan, is that the knowledge to be gained through one's analysis and their training is the knowledge of ignorance. Candidates are to learn what they do not know about themselves and about the analysands with whom they will eventually work.

The role of the formators in this process is to facilitate this knowledge of ignorance. "The candidate's training cannot be completed," argued Lacan (2007, p. 297), "without some action on the part of the master or masters who train him in this nonknowledge – failing which he will never be anything more than a robotic analyst." Without the gain of this knowledge, derived during one's analysis, a candidate will only ever be an analytical automaton, an analyst of artificial intelligence.

The acquisition of ignorance is akin to what Wang (2003, p. 101) referred to as "un-formation." The candidate approaches analytic formation with an existing sense of Imaginary identity based on years of lived experience. This identity (for the neurotic) must be put into question, unformed, deconstructed, to reach a position of ignorance. The source of true knowledge, the unconscious, must be brought to speech.

Hence, while one's personal psychoanalysis provides this education through experience, an institute is responsible for the formal transmission of techniques to work with speech. This is the linguistic dimension. As Tardits (2018, p. 93) described, "it is essential that [the candidate] be instructed in the knowledge and know-how of other practices of the letter." As Lacan (2007, p. 391) stated, "Such training would cover the distinction between the signifier and the signified" as first dictated by Ferdinand de Saussure, though Lacan traced as far back as St. Augustine.

To work with speech, one must have a foundation in various disciplines of the liberal arts. What future patients will speak about concerns their Symbolic place in the world, unique terms and turns of phrases the future analyst needs to have some familiarity with to work or play with them. Language fluency is important here. Cultural competency is another component of this dimension. One need only look to Lacan's seminars and the enormous width and depth of literature from which he pulled to create his lectures.

The technical dimension involves the techniques which the analyst uses during analysis. This dimension is therefore a clinical dimension. Diagnoses (neurosis, psychosis, and perversion) and their corresponding mechanisms (repression, foreclosure, and disavowal, respectively) need to be understood to know how to situate oneself as an analyst in a given analysis. Correct diagnosis then allows for the prudent use of interventions such as punctuation, scansion, and interpretation.

Between the focus of speech and techniques of analysis, Lacan (1981, p. 19) identified four concepts as "fundamental" to psychoanalysis: the unconscious, repetition, transference, and the drive. Analytic candidates learn these concepts (among many others) through their attendance at seminars, case conferences, study groups (what Lacan termed cartels, more below), and their own scholarship.

What is learned in the classroom is only understood through experience. Eventually, candidates begin clinical work with around two analysands under the supervision of more experienced analysts. The supervisor, in Lacanian work, is not an expert. As Leader (2010, p. 235) argued, "Supervision can be construed as a process designed to make the supervisee question what they are doing." As candidates work to apply theory, they are expected to understand and articulate how they decide to apply the theory they have learned to treatment.

Beyond the objective assessment of whether the candidate is facilitating psychoanalysis as was taught to them, there is also mentorship. As Moncayo (2006, p. 529) argued, "The supervisor has to help the supervisee find his or her own style, beyond imitation, identification, and compliance and beyond disavowal, defiance, and identification with the opposite."

Where all of this experience in formation leads for the candidate is a unique contribution to the school and psychoanalysis as a discipline. Lacan was opposed to the goals of regurgitation or mimicry in psychoanalytic training. Each candidate must be assessed on an individual basis as to how they understand their process of formation and what they want to do with that insight. The analyst is committed, if not called, to the continuation, evolution, and dissemination of psychoanalysis.

The End of Priestly Formation

There are two components to the end of priestly formation. First, the candidate petitions to become a deacon. This petition can occur at the conclusion of the configuration stage or during the vocational synthesis stage. It is deeply important that the initiative of the candidate is required to become a deacon. While the people in authority allow or deny the progression, it is the desire of the individual which drives priestly formation.

The diaconate is clearly distinguished from the priesthood. However, it "is not possible to admit a candidate to the diaconate in the face of doubts concerning his suitability for the priesthood" (USCCB, 2022, p. 74). Approval for the diaconate hinges on several factors. Two necessary steps include taking the *Oath of Fidelity* and the *Profession of Faith*. The candidate declares their fidelity to the teaching of the Church and submits their humble obedience to its authority.

In the vocational synthesis stage, the deacon completes a minimum six-month residence. "Rather than 'on-the-job training,' this stage is the living of a vocation as an ordained minister, because the diaconate is a new ontological and existential reality" (USCCB, 2022, p. 63). Something about the person who has progressed to this stage has changed not just in knowledge or even piety, but in their being.

The deacon is integrated into his specific parish and diocese. He is no longer set apart from the community but entwined into its daily life. The deacon is an "official representative and a public figure" and is primarily serving the community rather than being served or formed in the seminary (USCCB, 2022, p. 64). The new deacon is not expected to be fully confident in his new role but "works to overcome any human fears" (USCCB, 2022, p. 258).

After the vocational-synthesis stage is complete, the deacon seeks ordination as a priest. "He is to petition his diocesan bishop or major superior in writing to be ordained, expressing his free intention and permanent commitment" (USCCB, 2022, p. 74). Ordination is not a natural step automatically granted to someone who completes a checklist of requirements.

Annual evaluations during seminary are framed by the qualities prescribed in Canon Law for ordination to Holy Orders: "integral faith, right intention, requisite knowledge, good reputation, integral morals and proven virtues, and the requisite physical and psychological health" (USCCB, 2022, p. 73). While multiple formators contribute to the decision for readiness, the diocesan bishop must provide his "official call in the name of the Church on the basis of a moral certitude that is founded upon positive evidence proving the suitability of a candidate for Holy Order" (USCCB, 2022, p. 75). The deacon becomes a priest.

Formation does not end with ordination but enters a new and lifelong reality. The *PPF* uses the term "accompaniment" to describe the intention or ideal of the period immediately following ordination (USCCB, 2022, p. 162). The recommendations revolve around the facilitation of opportunities for the new priest to be known, by their bishop, the pastor under whom they serve, other new priests, and their parishioners.

Berg (2018) described why this period is so important. Not all goes well for new priests. "Within the first five years, a percentage of [new priests] fall into vocational crisis…In the majority of such cases, these men had wounds that they never disclosed or dealt with during their formation" (Berg, 2018, p. 13). Ordination does not provide any sort of protection against future struggle because the priest, like any other person, has new experiences which prompt their own unique questions. Discernment continues. Regardless, ordination, the formal end of priestly formation, is a joyous occasion for the new priest, their family, friends, and formators, and especially for their parish.

The End of Psychoanalytic Formation

While priestly formation involves the progression through distinct stages, psychoanalytic formation includes certain mechanisms or experiences which are at times concurrent, at times progressive. Personal analysis has already been discussed above. There are also the cartel and the pass, two experiences which (could) herald the end of formation.

Lacan described the cartel in his *Founding Act*. This study group consists of, ideally, four people, with a "plus one" to select and direct the topic of study. The intent was to guard against a hierarchical or authoritarian structure which would force students to acquiesce to a predetermined doctrine. The cartel, by contrast, produced knowledge, formative to the individual, the school, and psychoanalysis as a discipline.

Lacan's description and use of cartels was not without significant confusion, opposition, and misuse (Soler, 2013; Gallagher, 2018). To that extent, cartels fit into the general reception of Lacan's work. However, cartels continue to function today, and not just in training and formation but constitute an important part of the ongoing life of institutes and schools.

Lacan (1968, p. 7) wrote, "The end of a psychoanalysis, superfluously said to be training *(didactique)* is the effective passage from psychoanalysand to psychoanalyst." The dimension of desire is indicative of this transition from candidate to analyst. For Lacan, "the result of a training analysis ought to be comprehended in terms of the unconscious, more specifically in terms of unconscious desire" (Libbrecht, 1999, p. 75). The demand to become an analyst is transformed, over the course of one's analysis and training, into the desire of the analyst. "In the Lacanian

School, during the training of the analyst, the analyst's desire is formed and given shape" (Mathew & Hopkins, 2023, p. 5).

The analyst's desire is a particular kind of desire. It is not, for example, a desire to heal or cure. Nor is it a desire to teach or convince. Certainly, it is not to judge, if by judge one means in the moral realm (i.e., right and wrong, duty and obligation). "The analyst's desire abjures mastery: as a matter of principle, the analyst does not speak for the patient" (Wilson, 2020, p. xv). The analysand, who once perceived the analyst as the Subject Supposed to Know, comes to realize the analyst does not know, and must testify what they have come to know about their unconscious and psychoanalysis.

The desire of the analyst is an "unflagging desire for the patient to come to therapy, to put his or her experience, thoughts, fantasies, and dreams into words, and to associate to them" (Fink, 1997, p. 7). The analyst desires analysis. While the process for getting to this point in personal analysis is complex and involves many concepts not addressed in this chapter (e.g. traversing the fundamental fantasy), the analysand accepts their lack and seeks to position themselves into the role of analyst. The experiences of being an analysand and an analyst-in-training (through their control cases) contribute to this transformation.

The candidate must testify to this experience to witnesses. This is the first step in the procedure of the pass. The candidate, now termed the *passand*, speaks to two (at a minimum) *passers*. Then, the *passers* communicate what they learned about the *passand*'s experience in analysis to a jury. While it is not the same in every school, that jury is its own cartel. Should the cartel recognize the testimony, the *passand* is nominated to be an Analyst of the School (Lacan, 1968, p. 2).

Crucially, neither of these designations is required to be a psychoanalyst. As Lacan (1968, p. 1) argued, "the psychoanalyst derives his authorization only from himself." A candidate decides when their analysis has concluded and may practice analysis without these designations (though legal permission varies country to country). What these titles provide is an association to the School. These titles also come with significant responsibility to the School. The new analyst is responsible for the progress of the School.

If the *passer* is not nominated by the jury to be an Analyst of the School, in many cases, they are provided with feedback as to why. In general, the jury has determined there is more unconscious material for the candidate to address. Then, their work in personal analysis and the other components of formation continue until they decide again to seek the passage to become an analyst.

Just as the beginning of analysis is not equated with the physical entry into the consulting room, the end of analysis is not equated with the exit of the classroom or even the attainment of the title of Analyst of the School. At the end of analytic formation, Freud (1964b, p. 228) noted "the candidate is only a beginner and not yet a master. What is still needed must be acquired by practice and by an exchange of ideas in the psycho-analytical societies in which young and old members meet together." Formation continues.

Discussion

Through priestly formation, the candidate develops a sense of how everything works, fits together, within himself, within humanity, and within the whole of God's creation. The seminarian gains awareness of his place in the middle of the narrative with some knowledge of the beginning and end of the Christian life. The seminarian gains interior freedom and the skills necessary to facilitate this peace within his parish and wider world.

Through psychoanalytic formation, the candidate develops a sense of what is not working, what is broken, within himself, herself, or their self. There is a clarity that develops about their role and its limits. They recognize the analyst does not possess the knowledge they supposed they did in the beginning of their analysis. The candidate accepts this lack in themself in the face of the mystery of the unconscious.

Both the Church and Lacanians argue their training is not professional schooling or the attainment of knowledge but involves a change at the deepest level of being. "Formation, as the Church understands it, is not equivalent to a secular sense of schooling or, even less, of job training" (USCCB, 2022, p. 54). "The psychoanalytic institution is not a scientific society, nor a union to protect the rights of the psychoanalysts, although at times both may be needed." (Rodríguez, 2019, p. 122). The seminary and school are places where identity is formed to perform a specific role within a larger community.

Yet, priestly formation presumes a fundamental difference in the personal faith exploration of lay people and the professional faith of men discerning priestly vocation. Such a difference was the subject of debate in psychoanalysis between lay analysts and medically trained analysts. Lacan worked to diminish the difference between a training analysis and a therapeutic analysis. For Lacan, there is only one analytic process. Is there only one spiritual formation?

The requirements for admission to priestly formation are at times divorced from practical considerations or consequences. That is, the criteria are derived from doctrine rather than the lived experience of the priest and parish. For example, it is painfully obvious that Berg had not spoken to enough homosexual men to realize not all same-sex attracted 20-year-olds are emotionally turbulent, or that emotional turbulence can be part and parcel of early adulthood, or that rigid and moralistic messages contribute to such emotional turbulence. The final report from German Church authorities confirmed that homosexuality is not a risk factor for sexual abuse (Novotny, 2023, p. 114). There is no reason to prohibit gay men from seminary apart from significantly contested ideas about whether orientation constitutes sin.

In addition, the *PPF* questioned whether victims of sexual abuse are fit for priestly formation. Despite the sympathetic tenor, it is troubling that victims of the Church's abuse and cover up of that abuse are here singled out as potentially unfit for the clergy. Many seminarians were victims of clerical sexual abuse. Seeing them now as almost inherently unfit exacerbates their pain. The other actions mentioned in the *PPF* (abortion, self-harm, etc.) represent some of the worst suffering possible in life, even for perpetrators. The assumption implicit in these exclusionary criteria, that such people are unfit for priesthood, contradicts the longstanding tradition of the wounded healer beautifully outlined by Father Henri Nouwen (1972).

There is significant pressure for men to perform an image which meets expectations rather than genuinely grapple with the conflict in themselves and with the Church's teaching. While the guidance for formation insists on the need for honest deliberation and reflection on whether priestly formation is right for the individual, it potentially invites an unscrupulous performance to achieve the desired end of ordination. Criteria for admission must not be too rigid or numerous to distract from the fundamental factor: being called by God.

Gender is another important factor. During the recent Synod on Synodality, multiple study groups promoted the topic of the female diaconate. The Dicastery for the Doctrine of the Faith (previously, the Holy Office), censored this topic. The Synod, which was intended to be a unique opportunity for the Church to hear from its lay members, instead took this topic off the table (Wooden, 2024). Yet the debate over female ordination sidelines the question of masculinity. Masculinity is not self-evident and not exhausted by biological identification. The Church cannot hope to address the needs of gender by shelving it for another day. Psychoanalysis is uniquely capable of helping to facilitate this conversation.

Priestly formators should similarly consider whether and why their faith formation is different from the faith of their laypeople. If any psychoanalysis could result in the production of an analyst, any, shall we say, spiritual direction, could produce a clergyperson. Fewer and fewer men are inquiring into, let alone committing to, priestly formation. Rather than presuppose the production of a priest, the Church might find more success in promoting a broader process of formation for all Catholics.

Another important difference is the notion of progress. If the seminarian expresses a need for which long term therapy is recommended, they must leave the seminary. If they are not approved to progress to the next stage, they are advised to leave the seminary. The guidance is clear that seminary formation is not a treatment for spiritual or other illness but takes a healthy man to greater heights in his capacity to love, lead, and serve others.

This movement and progression make sense; after all, who would want a priestly candidate wracked with neurotic anxiety, affective immaturity, or financial irresponsibility? But the standard the guidance describes betrays a different conception of human nature compared to psychoanalysis and risks contradicting their own insistence of the lifelong nature of formation. This perspective is much too focused on ego development rather than wrestling with one's unconscious.

One of the reasons the Church applies such rigid and precise requirements for applicants to seminaries is the responsibility future priests hold for their parish communities. With all the downsides of the hierarchy of the Church, such a unified system also provides a clear purpose and places for the priests it forms.

Without suggesting that Lacanians develop their own magisterium of doctrinal authority, there is a question as to what the corresponding social body is for psychoanalysis, in its formation programs and later practices, and what universal responsibilities psychoanalysts hold. Lacan insisted on the ethics of psychoanalysis and yet this ethics has remained somewhat insulated in the profession.

Psychoanalysts, perhaps inspired by Lacan's own conflicts with authority, seem to accept too readily the inevitable splits and conflicts without any end in mind. One well-worn joke is that when there are two analysts in a city, there are three institutes. Much damage has been done as a result. Despite the humility analysis is presumed to instill in the future analyst, there remains an alluring idealization and grandiosity in the role and title of psychoanalyst. Institutes contribute to this image as they exercise significant subjectivity (and bias) when deciding who will be admitted to formation.

Psychoanalytic training would benefit from facilitating greater community between students and faculty and their institutes. As Baekeland (2019, p. 506) described, "Analysts work alone. Although we are with someone in a room, we are not really with someone. We cannot freely and fully be who we are with them." The desire of the analyst in the consulting room must be complemented by opportunities outside the consulting room for people to be together, across theoretical lines.

There are institutes, clinics, cartels, university departments, conferences, and congresses. What constitutes the psychoanalytic parish? Conceptualizing such a purpose and place would allow psychoanalytic ethics to be taken more seriously by the Church and the world at large. What is psychoanalysis for, besides the encounter in the consulting room? Service is typically construed as offering low fee sessions. That cannot be the sum total of the self-sacrifice to which psychoanalysts are committed. The ethics of psychoanalysis demands more.

References

Baekeland, C. (2019). How participating in an international community of psychoanalysts can offset local psychoanalytic institutes' insularities and enliven practice. *International Journal of Psychoanalysis*, 100(3): 505–517.

Barnes , M.W. (2022). Catholic seminarians on "real men", sexuality, and essential male inclusivity. *Religions*, 13: 352.

Berg, T. (2018). Getting formation right. *First Things*, December: 11–14.

Cullinan, E. (2019). Some thoughts on the future formation of priests. *The Furrow*, 70 (7/8): 414–418.

Drescher, J. (2008). A history of homosexuality and organized psychoanalysis. *The Journal of the American Academy of Psychoanalysis and Dynamic Psychiatry*, 36(3).

Dulle, C. (2024). The seminary today: How young priests are formed will impact the church for years to come. *America Magazine*, July/August: 18–23.

Fink, B. (1997). *A clinical introduction to Lacanian psychoanalysis: Theory and technique.* Harvard University Press.

Freud, S. (1964a). On psychotherapy. In J. Strachey (Ed. & Trans.), *The standard edition of the complete psychological works of Sigmund Freud*, Vol. 7 (pp. 255–268). (Original work published 1905)

Freud, S. (1964b). The question of lay analysis. In J. Strachey (Ed. & Trans.), *The standard edition of the complete psychological works of Sigmund Freud*, Vol. 20 (pp. 179–258). (Original work published 1926)

Friedman, R.C. & Downey, J.I. (1998). Psychoanalysis and the model of homosexuality as psychopathology: A historical overview. *The American Journal of Psychoanalysis*, 58(3): 249–270.

Gallagher, C. (2018). The founding act, the cartel and the riddle of the plus one. In L. Bailly, D. Lichtenstein, & S. Bailly (Eds.), *The Lacan Tradition* (pp. 75–95). Routledge.

Kohut, H. (1968). The evaluation of applicants for psychoanalytic training. *International Journal of Psychoanalysis*, 49: 548–554.

Lacan, J. (1949). Réglement et doctrine de la commission de l'enseignement déléguée par la sociéte psychanalytique de Paris. *Revue Française de Psychanalyse*, 13(3): 426–435.

Lacan, J. (1968). Proposition du 9 octobre 1967 sur le psychanalyste de l'Ecole. (R. Grigg, Trans.). *Scilicet*, 1: 14–30.

Lacan, J. (1981). *The four fundamental concepts of psychoanalysis.* (J-A. Miller, Ed.) (A. Sheridan, Trans.). W.W. Norton & Company.

Lacan, J. (2007). *Écrits: The first complete English edition.* (B. Fink, Trans.). W.W. Norton.

Leader, D. (2010). Some thoughts on supervision. *British Journal of Psychotherapy*, 26(2): 228–241.

Lewes, K., Young-Bruehl, E., Roughton, R., Magee, M., & Miller, D. (2008). Homosexuality and psychoanalysis I: Historical perspectives. *Journal of Gay & Lesbian Mental Health*, 12(4): 299–323.

Libbrecht, K. (1999). The original sin of psychoanalysis: On the desire of the analyst. In D. Nobus (Ed.), *Key concepts of Lacanian psychoanalysis.* Other Press.

Magee, M. & Miller, D. (1998). Homosexuality and psychoanalytic training. In M. Magee & D. Miller (Eds.), *Lesbian lives* (pp. 221–244). Routledge.

Mathew, D. & Hopkins, N. (2023). Training for the impossible? Induction and identity formation among trainee teachers and psychoanalysts. *Modern Psychoanalysis*, 47(1): 223–239.

Miller, J.A. (2003). *Contraindications to psychoanalytic treatment.* London Society of the New Lacanian School. https://londonsociety-nls.org.uk/wp-content/uploads/miller-jacques-alain_contraindications-to-psychoanalytical-treatment.pdf.

Moncayo, R. (2006). Lacanian perspectives on psychoanalytic supervision. *Psychoanalytic Psychology*, 23(3): 527–541.

Nouwen, H. (1972). *The wounded healer.* Image Books.

Novotny, S. (2023). Power versus ministry? Recent challenges for priestly formation in responding to the double crisis in the Catholic Church. *Journal of Moral Theology*, 12: 106–121.

Quinet, A. (1999). The functions of the preliminary interviews. *European Journal of Psychoanalysis*, 8–9.

Rodríguez, S.A. (2019). The psychoanalytic institution: teaching, ethics, refuge and solitude. *Analysis*, 22:119–126.

Sachs, H. (1947). Observations of a training analyst. *The Psychoanalytic Quarterly*, 16(2):157–168.

Selvam, S. (2019). "Moulding his personality": Personality change and formation to priesthood in the Catholic Church. *Journal of Spiritual Formation and Soul Care*, 12(2): 232–245.

Soler, C. (2013). The experience of the cartels of the pass of the 'Ecole de la Cause Freudienne.' (M. Williams & J. Holland, Trans.). *Analysis*, 18: 97–102.

Tardits, A. (2018). *The trainings of the psychoanalyst*. Routledge.

United States Conference of Catholic Bishops. (2022). *Program for Priestly Formation* (6th Ed). United States Conference of Catholic Bishops.

Wang, W.J. (2003). Bildung or the formation of the psychoanalyst. *Psychoanalysis and History*, 5(2): 91–119.

Wilson, M. (2020). *The analyst's desire: The ethical foundation of clinical practice (psychoanalytic horizons)*. Bloomsbury Academic.

Wooden, C. (2024). Vatican doctrinal chief tells synod it's not time for women deacons. *Catholic News Service.* https://www.usccb.org/news/2024/vatican-doctrinal-chief-tells-synod-its-not-time-women-deacons.

Chapter 8

The Name of the (Holy) Father

Towards a Synodal Discourse

On September 25, 2023, the Holy See published the responses of Pope Francis (2023) to five *dubia* he received from two Cardinals. *Dubia* is Latin for doubts. The Cardinals sought clarification on the Holy Father's interpretation and teaching of doctrine regarding the immutability of Divine Revelation, the blessing of same-sex unions, the influence of synodality on Church governance, the possibility of female ordination, and forgiveness as a human right.

Francis (2023, para. 8) stated:

> Dear Brothers, Although it does not always seem prudent to me to respond to questions directly addressed to my person, and it would be impossible to answer all of them, I have deemed it appropriate to do so in this case, given the proximity of the Synod.

This sentence contains many interesting elements, explored below, perhaps not evident on a surface-level reading. Francis was intentional in the discourse he used to respond to these Cardinals.

These *dubia* were not the first Pope Francis received during his papacy. Yet these *dubia* came from notable critics of his papacy, Cardinal Burke and Cardinal Brandmuller. These *dubia* therefore were not innocent doubts which sought edifying clarification but active interrogations of the sovereign authority of the Church.

This chapter explores the unique approach Pope Francis took to papal authority. He used a distinct and at times contradictory papal discourse. The psychoanalyst Jacques Lacan (1981) developed a theory of four discourses: master, university, hysteric, and analyst. Lacanian discourse is a method of understanding and working with language which impacts the Other. Discourse always involves an Other. This framework is used to interpret two moments in the papacy of Francis to determine strengths and weaknesses of his discourses and the conflict within the papacy itself to commit to any one discourse.

DOI: 10.4324/9781003485346-11

Lacanian Discourse

Lacan (1981) argued language usage occurs in a field of discourse which contributes to the development of the human subject. Because the unconscious is structured like a language, the language used contributes to the formation of the unconscious. "Language is the condition of the unconscious" (Lacan (1981, p. 41). This is one reason why diagnosis in Lacanian psychoanalysis is defined and determined by how the analysand uses language.

People choose their language to impact another person. All language is communicated with another person in mind, whether literally present or not. Therefore, discourse institutes a social bond. Lacan identified four possible discourses which institute four types of social bonds.

Discourse is not the same as identity. While someone may have the psychic structure of hysteria, they may not always use the hysteric's discourse (Fink, 2025). Discourse changes depending on the position an individual wants to use and the position in which they wish to place the other.

Lacan (1981) outlined four positions in discourse: agent, other, truth, and product or loss.

The agent is the person who is speaking, who addresses the other. Lacan (1981, p. 131) described the agent as "someone who is caused to act." The agent is also the one who is (covering) over truth. The truth is the motivation of the agent which the agent attempts to hide from the other. The other, who is addressed by the agent, produces something for the agent, the product of their work which they do not possess, hence it is a loss for the other. These components are displayed in a formula (Lacan (1981, p. 169; see also Clemans & Grigg, 2006, p. 3):

$$\frac{\text{agent}}{\text{truth}} \rightarrow \frac{\text{other}}{\text{product}}$$

Lacan then used symbols to represent four roles which occupy these positions in different ways. First is S_1: the master signifier. This is the signifier which does not associate with other signifiers. It is a role which stands alone. Lacan's "Name of the Father" is an example. For someone to say, "Because your father said so" is to employ a master signifier. As Fink (2025, p. 131) argued, "The master must be obeyed – not because we'll all be better off that way or for some other such rationale – but because he or she says so." The master signifier is a role of power.

Then there is S_2 which represents Symbolic knowledge, or what is already (unconsciously) known. As Lacan (1981, p. 33) put it, "knowledge that is not known." S_2 contains all other signifiers which S_1 uses to produce an outcome. S_2 is the existing signifying chain. As Evans (1996, p. 96) defined it, "Symbolic knowledge is knowledge of the truth about one's unconscious desire." This knowledge is distinct from so-called self-awareness, what people consciously think or *imagine* they know about themselves.

There is enjoyment in this image, what Lacan termed *jouissance,* which must be renounced in pursuit of the unconscious truth. This knowledge is not located within the mind but is an intersubjective relation because the unconscious is structured by the Other's discourse. It comes into being through speech.

The split subject in Lacanian psychoanalysis, the subject who is divided between their unconscious and conscious mind, is represented by the $ symbol (not the U.S. dollar), the S being the subject and the line representing the split or divide. As Lacan (1981, p. 177) said, "The subject's division is without doubt nothing other than the radical ambiguity that attaches itself to the very term, 'truth.'" The split subject can never fully know the truth about themselves because there is always some knowledge which remains unconscious.

Finally, there is the italicized letter *a.* This symbol represents the combination of Lacan's concept of object (*a*) and his concept of surplus *jouissance.* "The object *a* is what makes it possible to introduce a little bit of air into the function of *surplus jouissance*" (Lacan, 1981, p. 178). Surplus is the product of the work of S_2 which they do not possess for themselves, it is their loss, and as such, it is an imagined object which causes or drives their desire to obtain it (from another), thus continuing the work.

Each of these roles can occupy one position in the matrix provided above. The positions are unalterable while the roles move into different positions. Notice there is no arrow on the second line between truth and product. Lacan intentionally provided this blank. "Not only is there no communication, but there is something that acts as a block" (Lacan, 1981, p. 174). As is shown below, while any of the symbols can occupy any of the positions, "under no circumstances will production have a relationship to truth" (Lacan (1981, p. 174). Work does not produce truth.

With the positions and the roles described, the four different discourses can be understood.

The master's discourse places the master (signifier), S_1, in the position of agent, the dominant one. The other is occupied by S_2, the slave/worker/knowledge. The worker provides or produces obedience, *a*, to the master. "The master is unconcerned with knowledge: as long as everything works, as long as his or her power is maintained or grows, all is well" (Fink, 2025, p. 131). Obedience generates power in excess, that is, surplus. It reinforces the master's position. One might consider a billionaire capitalist. Their workers produce profit in excess of the needs of the business and CEO and far more than the person could ever spend. It is pure enjoyment.

$$\frac{S_1}{\$} \rightarrow \frac{S_2}{a}$$

The hidden truth is $, that the master is not all powerful or all-knowing but is, in fact, a lacking being not so different from the slave. They do not possess perfect business acumen or intelligence. They are not all knowing. The CEO is not so different from the janitor who cleans their office. Yet if this were to be known, the master would lose the power and money their position affords them. No one would want to work for them.

For the purposes of this chapter, the master of the Church, the pope, historically was situated in this position. The Name of the (Holy) Father was unquestioned power. Evangelization was the work of the Catholic worker whose knowledge was used to produce more Catholics (or reduce the number of non-Catholics) who conformed to the Law of the Church. More Catholics meant more money which meant more papal power. Certainly, cause was given over time for many to question the mastery of the pope. The doctrine of papal infallibility, not defined until the late nineteenth century, represented an attempt to have it both ways, to admit the pope's human nature and legitimize moments of divine power. Few popes have made use of that power since then.

Next is the university discourse. Starting with the roles and positions in the master's discourse, the symbols move counterclockwise. Now it is knowledge, S_2, which occupies the agent position. As Fink (2025, p. 132) described, "Systematic knowledge is the ultimate authority, reigning in the stead of blind will, and everything has its reason." This knowledge is systematic because it takes an authoritative stance to provide an explanation for everything. Nothing is a mystery, only something yet to be explained. This body of knowledge cannot be questioned.

$$\frac{S_2}{S_1} \rightarrow \frac{a}{\$}$$

S_2 addresses a, demanding that it fit into the explanations of its knowledge. The university, professor, or even the discipline of education itself, has a one directional dynamic with the student. The student is alienated from true knowledge. They can never learn enough. They remain dependent on the university. More students, unknowing subjects, are produced, represented by $\$$. The S_2 needs to keep hidden that its truth is S_1, that its supposed objective knowledge is driven by the master signifier. The university is at the service of the master who wants the students to remain within the system. If the students knew this truth, they would rebel against the university. Lacan did not simply theorize this from a void, he gleaned insight from the significant protests in France in the 1960s.

To consider the topic raised in the previous chapter, priestly formation, there is a question regarding to what extent seminaries function using the discourse of the university. Do they encourage the seminarians to pursue a genuine science, that is, pursuit of truth which may lead to profound questions of power, or do seminaries demand seminarians adhere to an objective, complete knowledge which rationalizes their position and supports the power of the Magisterium and the Church? The answer is bound to be dependent on specific schools. The subject admitted and later produced by the seminary gives important clues.

Turning counterclockwise again, the diagram becomes the discourse of the analyst and, for Lacan, the basis on which psychoanalytic treatment must occur. The agent is the cause of desire, *a*, which addresses the split subject, $. "The analyst plays the part of pure desirousness (pure desiring subject), and interrogates the subject in his or her division, precisely at those points where the split between conscious and unconscious shows through" (Fink, 2025, p. 135). What the agent/analyst wants from the other, the analysand, the $, is the master signifier, S_1, which is at the root of their symptoms.

$$\frac{a}{S_2} \rightarrow \frac{\$}{S_1}$$

Lacan taught that on the side of the analyst, the literal left side of the diagram, is knowledge, S_2.

> It's on his side that there is S_2, that there is knowledge – whether he acquires this knowledge through listening to his analysand, or whether it is already acquired, locatable knowledge, which at a certain level can be limited to analytic know-how.
>
> (Lacan, 1981, p. 35)

What Lacan meant is that the analyst has learned various things about the analysand (their history, their family, their job, etc.) and the analyst has their knowledge of psychoanalytic theory and technique. With this technique, the analyst can make use of the knowledge of the analysand to interrogate the analysand for the truth of the master signifier. With the analyst as agent, the analyst pushes the analysand to keep working, keep talking, until the unconscious truth is spoken. It is up to the analysand to decide when that process must stop and the analyst as *a* becomes a loss.

Finally, there is the discourse of the hysteric. Turning the diagram again, the agent is occupied by $, the split subject. The $ as agent interrogates the other, S_1, the master signifier. "The hysteric goes at the master and demands that he or she show his or her stuff, prove his or her mettle by producing something serious by way of knowledge" (Fink, 2025, p. 133). As described above, the master is a role of unquestioned authority and knowledge. For the hysteric to question the master is akin to saying, "prove it!" The hysteric does not believe the master can prove it and is pushing the master to admit they lack the knowledge and power they claim to hold. This enjoyment, S_2, is therefore located under the master, S_1. Meanwhile, the hysteric as agent covers over and does not want others to see they themselves are a lacking, divided subject, looking for the lost object, *a*.

$$\frac{\$}{a} \rightarrow \frac{S_1}{S_2}$$

Lacan (1981, p. 23) provocatively argued "What leads to knowledge is – allow me to justify this in the more or less long term – the hysteric's discourse." The master has no need of knowledge so long as his power remains intact. The university does not want knowledge insofar as it wants others to believe it already has it. The hysteric wants knowledge. "It is around the symptom that the hysteric's discourse is situated and ordered" (Lacan, 1981, p. 43). The hysteric poses their symptom to the other, the analyst, and demands they explain it. This prompts the analyst to recognize their limit of knowledge and do their own work in the innovation of theory. Freud certainly found himself doing so due to his work with hysteria (Fink, 2025, p. 134).

None of these discourses should be seen as better or worse than the others. To think that there is a right or correct discourse is to misunderstand Lacan's intention with this matrix. While Lacan argued psychoanalysis requires the analyst to use the analyst's discourse to produce the intended change, this does not mean that the other discourses are useless. As described above, the hysteric's discourse has significantly aided the development of psychoanalysis. Besides, in the conversation in session, only the analyst situates themself with the analyst's discourse and in so doing, pushes the analysand into the hysteric's discourse.

Each discourse has its utility. It is a question of using the discourses in the appropriate context dependent on the desired outcome. The remainder of this chapter will explore in what ways and in what circumstances Pope Francis and his interlocutors used these discourses and to what effect. Synodality was an important signifier for Pope Francis which had its strengths and weaknesses. Doing so will help elucidate motivations for the praise and the criticism Pope Francis received during his papacy. Such an analysis implicates everyone in the dialogue and resists the simplistic reduction to a progressive/conservative divide. In the end, this chapter argues that Lacanian discourse analysis can strengthen the synodal way of the Church.

Cardinal Hysteria and Papal Analysis

The four discourses of Lacan help to illuminate the complicated exchange between Pope Francis and the Cardinals described at the start of the chapter. The term *dubia*, or doubts, already suggests the discourse of the hysteric. Their refrain across each doubt, "It is asked…", sought knowledge from the master whom they doubted possessesed the knowledge and authority.

These *dubia* did not arise out of nowhere but formalized criticisms Pope Francis had received since the beginning of his papacy. The Cardinals sought to pin him down in positions of knowledge they could then reveal as lacking (in relation to Church doctrine).

While the Cardinals used the hysteric's discourse, Pope Francis appeared to sidestep their appeal to a master and instead replied with the discourse of the analyst. While Francis's (2023, para. 8) opening greeting, "Dear brothers," suggested a fraternal bond, the next sentence introduced ambiguity: "It does not always seem prudent to me to respond to questions directly addressed to my person." Such a sentence could be spoken by a psychoanalyst! After all, directly responding to a personal question would be to use the master's discourse, or to presume that one really is the subject who knows.

Dubia have historically been addressed and responded to by Vatican officials in charge of various departments, "the Dicastery for the Doctrine of the Faith, the Dicastery for Divine Worship and the Discipline of the Sacraments, and especially the Dicastery for Legislative Texts" because these staff members are considered the authorities with the expertise to respond (Bunson, 2023, para. 5). It is rare for the pope to receive *dubia* addressed to him.

Again, to address Pope Francis, the Cardinals positioned themselves as the dominant agent $ who challenged the master S_1. They wanted Francis to respond using the master's discourse. Francis resisted this position. Francis (2023, para. 8) recognized the limit of that discourse, writing, "It would be impossible to answer all of [those questions]."

In other words, Pope Francis was aware that the master does not possess all knowledge, therefore he stated at the outset, in this discourse, he would not claim that mantle. This was a tricky position for the pope of all people to maintain, positioned as he was at the head of an organization with billions of members which claims authoritative, divine truth.

The rest of the opening sentence read, "I have deemed it appropriate to do so in this case, given the proximity of the Synod" (Francis, 2023, para. 8). Francis indicated his response was not given to satisfy the *jouissance* of the Cardinals. To respond to them after he indicated he does not often respond to these questions from others might suggest he finds them, as Lacan might put it, precious. Francis dismissed them as the cause of his desire to respond.

Instead, Pope Francis pointed to the "proximity of the Synod" as the cause of his desire to respond. The Synod was the Synod on Synodality, which Francis initiated and facilitated between 2021–2024 (General Secretariat of the Synod, 2021). His reference to the Synod as the cause of and reason for his response to the Cardinals was significant. First, in referring to the Synod, Francis tied the Cardinals' questions to the larger process of the Synod.

Some background: a synod in the Catholic Church was historically a meeting of clergy members to solve contemporary problems faced by the Church. "In the course of church history, the main task of synods was the discernment for the common preservation of the Christian faith in threatening situations" (Mayer, 2020, p. 206). Cardinals and Bishops would gather and respond to these questions and dictate their answers to the lay faithful.

Pope Francis radically altered this norm by his inclusion of laypeople, including women, into the Synod on Synodality. Some bishops and cardinals took issue with this change, as it made their role no more significant than a layperson. When Francis tied the Cardinals' questions to the synod process, he indicated his response to them was grounded in his synodal perspective which saw all members of the church as having a voice in the direction of the church.

Second, his reference to the synod at the outset is also significant because the third *dubium* questioned the *authoritative* status of synodality in relation to the authority of the Magisterium. The Cardinals doubted whether synodality could be "constitutive" of Church governance. Pope Francis indicated synodality *authorized* his response to the Cardinals. In other words, the two Cardinals would not have received the response/knowledge they sought without synodality.

The Cardinals did not just ask questions, they also insisted on what they already knew. They referenced the Catechism, documents issued by the Second Vatican Council, an apostolic letter authored by Pope St. John Paul II, the Book of Exodus, and a letter of St. Paul to question Pope Francis. Their questions sought yes or no answers.

Can divine revelation change? Can the Church bless same-sex unions when revealed doctrine says no? Is synodality the "supreme regulatory criterion" for Church governance (*dubium* three)? Are the teachings of the Second Vatican Council and John Paul II still valid? Is contrition still required for absolution?

These questions are reminiscent of the Pharisees when they challenged Jesus in the New Testament. Why do your disciples eat on the Sabbath? (Matt. 12:2, New Revised Standard Version: Catholic Edition); Is it lawful to cure on the Sabbath? (Matt. 12:10) Who gave you this authority? (Matt. 21:23); Why do your disciples not follow tradition? (Mark 7:5)? The Pharisees tried to seduce Jesus with their "knowledge" that he was "truthful" but asked, is it lawful to pay taxes to the emperor, or not? (Matt. 22:17). The discourse of the hysteric is also the discourse of the Pharisees.

How did Jesus respond? Rather than provide direct answers to their questions, Jesus asked questions in return. "Have you not read what David did when he and his companions were hungry?" (Matt. 12:3); "Will you not lay hold of [a sheep] and lift it out [on the Sabbath]?" (Matt. 12:11); "Did the baptism of John come from heaven, or was it of human origin?" (Matt. 21:25); "Whose head is this, and whose title?" (Matt. 22:20)?

Jesus also pointed out contradictions, told ambiguous parables, and performed miracles which drew attention to the holes in the Pharisees' knowledge of themselves and of the law. Jesus did not respond with yes or no answers but provided interventions which provoked the Pharisees (and others who listened to these exchanges, especially his disciples) to think. Jesus made use of the analyst's discourse.

This comparison between the Cardinals who authored the *dubia* and the Pharisees in the New Testament is not meant to malign the Cardinals. As stated above, the hysteric's discourse can lead to important advances in knowledge. The Pharisees' questions prompted significant opportunities for Jesus to teach key lessons to his followers. Without these exchanges, Christian doctrine today would lack significant knowledge.

Pope Francis made similar use of the analyst's discourse in his response to the Cardinals. When the Cardinals asked whether divine revelation can be reinterpreted despite its immutability, Francis (2023) responded, "The answer depends on the meaning you give to the word 'to reinterpret'" (answer 1a). He took a term which the Cardinals presumed to define and questioned it.

He then took their knowledge of Vatican II and created a tension: there is immutability attributed to divine origin, and interpretation within human limitations. There is a need for maturation. To paraphrase, Pope Francis asked the Cardinals, are not humans (i.e. the Cardinals) limited in their understanding and always in need of further maturation and growth?

To the second question regarding blessing same-sex unions, Pope Francis singled out the term marriage and essentially made it a master signifier. Marriage, he said, does not refer to any other meaning, it "has an essential constitution that is unique; as a result, it requires an exclusive name that is not applicable to other realities" (answer 2b). Marriage is a Church-sanctioned union between a man and a woman.

Does this not give the Cardinals the knowledge they sought? Perhaps. But Pope Francis then stated that marriage is not the only form of union. Through his introduction of the master signifier marriage, he problematized the signifier union.

With reference to Pope St. John Paul II, Pope Francis (2023) then challenged the Cardinals' knowledge of blessing. "When one asks for a blessing, one is expressing a petition for God's assistance, a plea to live better, and confidence in a Father who can help us live better" (answer 2e). Why should a same-sex couple, pleading to live better, not receive this blessing?

Again, Pope Francis resisted the discourse of the master. His answer, he warned them, should not become a rule. Even more to the point, "Canon Law should not and cannot cover everything, nor should the Episcopal Conferences claim to do so with their various documents and protocols, since the life of the Church flows through many channels besides the normative ones" (Francis, 2023, answer 2g). It is the duty of each pastor to discern the knowledge which would support each parishioner. Francis essentially told the Cardinals, get back to work.

The third question concerned synodality and governance. Pope Francis (2023) had previously described synodality as a "constitutive dimension of the Church" (*dubium* three). Yet the Synod of Bishops (which now includes lay people), the Cardinals wrote, "is merely an advisory body to the Pope" (*dubium* three). How, then, can synodality coexist with the "supreme and full authority of the Church" exercised by the Pope and the Magisterium? The Cardinals attempted to tie their authority to that of the papacy. If Francis diminished their authority, he would thereby diminish the authority of the papacy.

Pope Francis again did not respond directly to the question. He stated, "with these *dubia* you express your need to participate, to express your opinion freely, and to collaborate, and thereby you are invoking a form of 'synodality' in the exercise of my ministry" (answer 3a). He reflected back to them that with their questions, they expressed a lack in themselves and desire for accompaniment, to journey together with him. This expression is a manifestation of synodality. The Cardinals asked whether their authority is challenged by synodality and Francis confronted them with the reality that synodality provided them the tools to clarify their authority.

The fourth question concerned the difference between the priesthood of the faithful and the ordained priesthood available to select men (and not women). The Cardinals wanted a definitive answer as to whether the doctrine which bestows the priesthood only to men can ever be opened for debate.

Pope Francis first challenged their idea that one priesthood is superior to the other. "Both forms of priesthood," he stated, "illuminate and support each other" (Francis, 2023, answer 4a). Thus, women are not less than men if they do not have the opportunity to receive priestly ordination. Francis again appealed to St. John Paul II to note that ordination is about function, not value. The priesthood is about service to, not "domination" over, others.

This dynamic of service is beautifully illustrated in a scene in Paolo Sorrentino's *The New Pope* (2020). During the season, nuns living within the Vatican protested their harmful treatment by the resident priests. Fueled by feminist ideas about equality, the nuns petitioned the Pope to hear their ideas about how to become equal to the priests.

The fictional Pope Pius XII (played by Jude Law) challenged their idea of equality as being too tied to secular philosophy. Religious life in the Church, he reminded them, involves too much mystery that cannot be resolved by the world. He questioned why they sought equality to priests who had, in his estimation, moved "too close to civil society" (Sorrentino et al., 2020). He went on:

> It is not a matter of extending to you sisters the rights and privileges of the priests, but rather of extending to the priests the duties and the privations of you nuns. This is the only equality that is truly feasible in the Church.
>
> (Sorrentino et al., 2020)

The Church teaches equality in humility, not promotion.

In daily life, "The priests must do your laundry, just as you do theirs. They must look, within themselves, to find your grace, your generosity, your intelligence, and your love" (Sorrentino et al., 2020). Ordination to the priesthood does not confer wholeness on the man. It grants him certain authorities and responsibilities, but it also comes with lack. Priests need nuns, they need women, for qualities and knowledge they lack.

Pope Francis would have appreciated this scene. Women, Francis (2023) told the dubious Cardinals, "need…to participate in various ways in the leadership of the Church" (answer 4b). The Cardinals wanted a definitive declaration against female ordination. What they received instead was a declaration that women are needed in Church leadership.

As for ordination, Francis (2023) said, "let us recognize that a clear and authoritative doctrine on the exact nature of a 'definitive declaration' has not yet been fully developed" (answer 4c). The Cardinals asked for a type of papal declaration that does not exist in Canon Law. Francis did not take the opportunity to suddenly create it. Again, he sent the Cardinals back to work.

The final *dubium* asked Pope Francis (2023) whether contrition is necessary for absolution, given his assertion that "forgiveness is a human right" (*dubium* five). Francis did not deviate from his discourse. He stated that the sacrament of reconciliation is not conducted on the basis of "mathematics." Confession and absolution are not formulas with static variables. Repentance is not a master signifier, "there are many ways to express repentance" (answer 5b). In crystal clear terms, Francis stated, "We are not masters but humble stewards of the Sacraments" (answer 5a).

The "we" is not a "royal we." Had Pope Francis stated, "*you* are not masters," he would have used the master's discourse, and thereby encouraged the Cardinals in their hysteric attempt to undermine his authority. He stated "we must learn" to provide unconditional love (Francis, 2023). By including himself in the lack of mastery and the need to learn, Pope Francis again rejected the master's discourse and insisted there was joint work to be done.

Returning to the matrix of the hysteric's discourse, the Cardinals, with their questions of Pope Francis, placed themselves in the position of agent. The agent covers (over) the truth. For the hysteric as agent, the truth is object *a*. Fink (2025, p. 134) argued, "The truth of the hysteric's discourse, its hidden motor force, is the real."

The Real, one of the Lacanian registers of human subjectivity, is a complex concept. To put it too simply, the Real is an experience of reality which cannot be articulated in language. In the matrix, for the Real to be in the position of truth, means it is blocked from symbolic knowledge, S_2.

For the hysteric, and for the Cardinals, they must cover this black hole and act as if full knowledge is possible because it is that possibility which makes the Master, and his questioning, tenable. Paradoxically, this means that hysteric discourse must always have a master to address. The hysteric might succeed in "castrating" an individual as master, but they will need to find another master to address or else be confronted with the Real.

The Cardinals were not successful in their attempt to show the Pope as master was lacking. If they were, their position as agent would have collapsed. Cardinals need a Pope to exist. Yet even if they were successful, there is always another pope to step into the role. This continuity of the Catholic master introduces another motivation. There is, perhaps, a fantasy which drives the desire to castrate the master; to become the master of all knowledge. Protestantism is not exempt from this outcome, for while it rejected the pope as master, it created several thousand masters in its denominations.

One cardinal (typically, though not as a rule) can become the pope. When the seat of Peter is vacant (through death), a cardinal who uses the discourse of the hysteric has an opportunity to step into a role through which he imagines he can use the discourse of the master to accumulate more power. Yet he would learn, as Pope Francis seemed to know, that whatever that image of wholeness might be, is inherently lacking. The need to cover the Real of what is not working repeats.

That lesson was not learned by some brother cardinals. The following year, an anonymous letter was published in an Italian newspaper which criticized Pope Francis for being too ambiguous on doctrine (i.e. not using the master's discourse enough) while also being too authoritarian in Church governance (i.e. too much discourse of the master) (Giangravé, 2024). Unlike the *dubia*, this letter did not include questions and was not addressed to Pope Francis. This author had evidently resigned themselves that Pope Francis would not succumb to being the unmasked master.

Instead, this letter was addressed to other cardinals in view of the inevitable future conclave to choose a new pope. The discourse was no longer hysteric. The letter identified successes and shortcomings of Francis's papacy. It instructed other cardinals to prepare themselves for the future conclave. Though Francis was not castrated, resigned, or yet dead, the author of this letter decided to act as if Francis were. They acted as if there were no master.

They communicated full knowledge about the pros and cons of Francis's papacy, and they knew what cardinals needed to do to pick the best candidate for pope. In other words, they used the university discourse to get students (voting cardinals) to adhere to their knowledge. Doing so covered over their truth, their motivation, which was for that position and power of master.

The Synod on Synodality

Shortly after the Vatican published Pope Francis's responses to the *dubia*, he presided over the final session of the Synod on Synodality in Vatican City from October 4–29, 2023. Francis announced the beginning of the Synod in 2021. Francis (2021) insisted that the word synodal not be considered "yet another description or definition of the Church." That is, synodality was not one signifier among many, but a master signifier for the Church.

As such, its meaning extended back to the Acts of the Apostles, to the beginning of the Church. What started in Acts was a journey, not merely an institution. Members of the church, whether clergy or lay, accompanied one another on this journey, where no role is more important than any other.

This journey was initiated or prompted by "restlessness" in the Augustinian sense. For Pope Francis (2021), "This is essential: if Christians do not feel a deep inner restlessness, then something is missing. That inner restlessness is born of faith; it impels us to consider what it is best to do, what needs to be preserved or changed." Francis turned faith on its head: a Christian is not standing still in peace, but restless and on the move. The end is God, in the new heavens and new earth.

Those on the journey needed to be aware "this may mean setting out, changing course, leaving behind certain ideas that hold us back and prevent us from setting out and walking together" (Francis, 2021). Importantly, Francis noted that the Church is not a substitute taking the place of Jesus after his ascension. That role is filled by the Holy Spirit.

Pope Francis was aware of resistance to change. With reference to the composer Gustav Mahler, Francis asked, "What are you more inclined to do: guard the ashes of the Church, in other words, your association or group, or keep the fire burning?" It is not irrelevant that Mahler met with Sigmund Freud to address many psychological concerns; primarily, he wanted to "face himself" (Steinberg, 1999, p. 865). The synodal church faces itself in dialogue with the whole church.

Pope Francis outlined a multistep process. The first phase was the "consultation of the people of God" (General Secretariat of the Synod, 2021). This phase began with the diocesan stage. Every parish in every diocese was asked to facilitate meetings for its members to answer two guiding questions: "How does this journeying together allow the Church to proclaim the Gospel in accordance with the mission entrusted to Her" and "What steps does the Spirit invite us to take in order to grow as a synodal Church?" (General Secretariat of the Synod, 2021). The people, as sheep, "have their own 'sense of smell'" for "finding new paths for the journey, or for finding the road when the way is lost" (Francis, 2021).

The answers to these questions were collected by the diocese and the diocese held its own sessions to discuss the reports. The reports were then synthesized into a diocesan report, and, in the United States, all of the diocesan reports were synthesized into one national report. Following the diocesan and national stages, each continent assembled to facilitate the same process.

The final U.S. report included a section titled "Enduring Wounds" (USCCB, 2022, p. 5). These wounds included the continued pain caused by the sexual abuse and cover up of sexual abuse in the Church, the suffering caused by COVID-19, polarization in the Church, and marginalization. The latter wound included two groups. First, people marginalized by a "lack of power," such as the poor, immigrants, disabled, and incarcerated individuals (USCCB, 2022, p. 6).

Second, people marginalized by "circumstances in their own lives are experienced as impediments to full participation in the life of the Church" (USCCB, 2022, p. 6). The report included in this category "members of the LGBT+ community, persons who have been divorced or those who have remarried without a declaration of nullity, as well as individuals who have civilly married but who never married in the Church" (USCCB, 2022, p. 6). This second group of marginalized people experiencing enduring wounds and how to respond to their needs "surfaced in every synthesis" (USCCB, 2022, p. 6). These were issues Catholics in every diocese of the United States wanted discussed at the Synod.

The second phase, the "discernment of the pastors," included the first session of the assembly in Vatican City, the period between the first and second sessions, and the second assembly (General Secretariat of the Synod, 2021). In addition to the bishops, 70 non-bishops (lay men and women as well as religious men and women), were selected to participate and vote on the final documents. In total, there were 400 participants and 370 voting participants (Cernuzio, 2023).

Between the first and second sessions, Pope Francis initiated the creation of 10 study groups separate from the synod assemblies to discuss contentious issues which arose during the first session. These topics included female leadership in the church (such as the diaconate) and the inclusion of LGBT+ people in the life of the Church. Francis argued these topics needed "further study" and were excluded from the agenda at the second assembly (Wooden, 2024).

While most of these study groups produced summary videos for the assembly participants, the study group for women ordination did not do so. This study group, led by Cardinal Víctor Manuel Fernández, prefect of the Dicastery for the Doctrine of the Faith, determined that the question of female ordination was not "mature" for discussion at the synod (Wooden, 2024).

While lay Catholics across the United States (and many other countries) wanted this issue to be discussed, Cardinal Fernández said no. The final report of the Synod, authored by Pope Francis, stated, "the question of women's access to diaconal ministry remains open. This discernment needs to continue" (2024, p. 22). The final report did not use LGBT+ terminology or refer to that community by name.

These study groups were scheduled to submit their final reports on June 30, 2025. However, an extension was provided until December 31, 2025 (Brockhaus, 2025). It is now up to Pope Leo XIV to receive these reports and use their guidance as he makes decisions for the Church moving forward. The final report authored by Pope Francis (2024) was declared magisterial and "must be accepted" and implemented by the Church.

Synodal Discourse and its Limits

The overview above was brief and did not explore in detail each facet of the Synod process. There are many documents and speeches worth in depth review. There were important and groundbreaking conclusions which emerged from the Synod. While the assemblies are complete and the final report was published, synodality remains a key signifier for the Church. Pope Leo XIV has stated as such (Watkins, 2025).

However, the purpose of this chapter, much like the function of psychoanalysis, is to examine what did not work, what did not go well. Using Lacan's discourse theory, what sort of discourses were used in the Synod, and were those discourses effective?

At the start, much as Pope Francis did in his response to the cardinals, he appeared to use the discourse of the analyst. In his position as agent and cause of desire, he asked the other(s), the bishops, members of religious orders, and lay men and women, to speak about their perception of their symptoms and their desire for the Church. These others are represented in the matrix as $\$$, they are divided, between and within themselves. To simplify the matrix:

$$\frac{\text{Pope } (a)}{S_2} \rightarrow \frac{\text{Church } (\$)}{S_1}$$

The Pope and the Church are in their respective position as agent and other. What are the roles in the positions underneath them in the analyst's discourse? S_2 is knowledge that the analyst uses in interrogating the other. In this application, the knowledge under the Pope is all of the signifying chain spoken during the diocesan stage and carried forward into the various reports which led to the agenda for the first assembly.

Under the Church as other is the master signifier, what the Pope as analyst is presumed to want the Church to speak though it is unconscious to the Church. All other signifiers, for example, ordination, homosexuality, gender, poverty, immigration, emanate from the master signifiers. This is complicated, as millions of people contributed to the documents the Holy Father reviewed. Regardless, the matrix is now complete:

$$\frac{\text{Pope } (a)}{\text{Reports } (S_2)} \rightarrow \frac{\text{Church } (\$)}{\text{Product/Loss } (S_1)}$$

Pope Francis initiated the Synod and through the first assembly facilitated the discourse as an analyst. The Church was put to work to speak! However, the Church/other spoke of topics during the first assembly which the pope/analyst did not accept. Francis did not purely desire as the analyst must do. Inevitably, the pope, unlike an analyst, had a personal and professional stake in the outcome. Francis had opinions about what needed to be discussed and what needed to be delayed for another time.

The displacement of certain controversial topics to study groups, which lacked transparency and inclusion into the final report, was not an analytic act. Pope Francis, while he intended to welcome any and all speech in the sincere hope of addressing the unconscious roots of the Church's problems, used the discourse of the university. He knew what the Church should and should not speak about, what the Church was ready or mature enough to discuss. He backed away from the other's desire.

$$\frac{\text{Pope } (S_2)}{\text{truth } (S_1)} \rightarrow \frac{\text{Church } (a)}{\text{Obedience } (\$)}$$

Pope Francis then permitted the Church in the second assembly to speak about what he and his select group of cardinals determined was best for the Church. The product was obedience to remain within this restricted dialogue. The master signifier was now under Francis, with the hidden motivation to retain power with the excess pleasure of a unified Church.

An alternative interpretation of the shift in discourse would be to see Pope Francis as using the master's discourse. In this view, Francis was the master (S_1) who addressed the Church other as knowledge (S_2) to produce the excess pleasure (*a*) which continued the work of the Synod and sustained him as *the* synodal pope, while he hid his truth: he was divided and conflicted about what to do about these contemporary issues.

$$\frac{\text{Pope } (S_1)}{\text{Truth } (\$)} \rightarrow \frac{\text{Church } (S_2)}{\text{Synod } (a)}$$

Regardless of which application of Lacan's discourses is correct, one shared conclusion emerges: the Holy Father cannot sustain the discourse of the analyst. Synodality is an essential element of the Church and is vital for the Church to keep the flame alive a la Mahler. Synodality is best facilitated through the discourse of the analyst. What Pope Francis failed to realize is that even in his role as the sovereign pontiff sets him apart from all others, he remained part of the other, the Church.

The pope cannot effectively inhabit the role of analyst in the discourse of the analyst. Indeed, no one who claims to be a member of the Catholic Church can inhabit that role. If the true spirit of synodality is to be facilitated in future synods, the analytic discourse must include people who are not within the role of the other. The role of analyst must be filled by a non-Catholic, someone who can maintain the psychoanalytic ethical position of helping the other speak their unconscious desire.

References

Brockhaus, H. (2025, July 8). Vatican's synod office postpones reports on controversial issues. EWTN Vatican. https://www.ewtnvatican.com/articles/vaticans-synod-office-postpones-reports-on-controversial-issues-5875.

Bunson, M. (2023, October 2). Answering the doubts: What are 'dubia'? *National Catholic Register*. https://www.ncregister.com/cna/answering-the-doubts-what-are-dubia.

Cernuzio, S. (2023, April 26). Synod: Laymen and laywomen eligible to vote at General Assembly. *Vatican News*. https://www.vaticannews.va/en/vatican-city/news/. 2023–2004/synod-synodality-general-assemblies-laypeople-eligible-vote.html.

Clemans, J. & Grigg, R. (2006). Introduction. In J. Clemans & R. Grigg (Eds.), *Jacques Lacan and the other side of psychoanalysis: Reflections on Seminar XVII*. Duke University Press.

Evans, D. (1996). *An introductory dictionary of Lacanian psychoanalysis*. Routledge.

Fink, B. (2025). *The Lacanian subject: Between language and jouissance.* Princeton University Press.

Francis (2021). *Address of His Holiness Pope Francis to the faithful of the diocese of Rome. The Holy See. Vatican City.* https://www.vatican.va/content/francesco/en/speeches/2021/september/documents/20210918-fedeli-diocesiroma.html.

Francis (2023). *"Dubia" of two cardinals (10 July 2023) and "respuestas" of the Holy Father "a los dubia propuestos por dos cardenales" (11 July 2023). Dicasterium Pro Doctrina Fidei.* https://www.vatican.va/roman_curia/congregations/cfaith/documents/rc_con_cfaith_risposta-dubia-2023_en.html#.

Francis (2024). *For a synodal church: Communion, participation, mission. Final document. XVI General Assembly of the Synod of Bishops.* https://www.synod.va/content/dam/synod/news/2024-10-26_final-document/ENG—Documento-finale.pdf.

General Secretariat of the Synod. (2021). What is the synod about?https://www.synod.va/en/the-synod-on-synodality/what-is-the-synod-about.html.

Giangravé, C. (2024, March 1). Anonymous cardinals criticize Pope Francis as 'autocratic, vindictive' in new letter. *Religion News Service.* https://www.americamagazine.org/faith/2024/03/01/anonymous-letter-pope-francis-cardinals-247413/.

Lacan, J. (1981). *The other side of psychoanalysis. The Seminar of Jacques Lacan: Book XVII.* (J.A. Miller, Ed.) (R. Grigg, Trans.). W.W. Norton & Company.

Mayer, A.C. (2020). "For a synodal church": Equipping the Catholic Church on her way into the third millennium. *Louvain Studies*, 43: 205–214.

Sorrentino, P. (Writer & Director), Contarello, U. (Writer), & Bises, S. (Writer). (2020, January 31). Season 1, Episode 8 [TV Series episode]. In L. Mieli, M. Gianani, R. Neri, E. Recchia, P. Sorrentino, J. Law, C. Benjo, C. Scotta, S. Arnal, J. Roures, J. Méndez, N. Hartmann, S. Rovai, & D. Bertoni (Executive Producers). *The New Pope.* The Apartment Pictures; Wildside; Haut et Court TV; Mediapro; Sky Studios.

Steinberg, S. (1999). Tragic absurdity in the music of Gustav Mahler. *Psychoanalytic Review*, 86: 853–875.

United States Conference of Catholic Bishops. (2022). *National synthesis of the People of God in the United States of America or the Diocesan Phase of the 2021–2023 Synod.* https://www.usccb.org/resources/US%20National%20Synthesis%202021-2023%20Synod.pdf.

Watkins, D. (2025, June 26). Pope: Synodality is an attitude that helps Church foster communion. *Vatican News.* https://www.vaticannews.va/en/pope/news/2025-06/pope-leo-xiv-council-synod-church-synodality-communion.html.

Wooden, C. (2024, October 4). Vatican doctrinal chief tells synod it's not time for women deacons. *Catholic News Service.* https://www.usccb.org/news/2024/vatican-doctrinal-chief-tells-synod-its-not-time-women-deacons.

Chapter 9

Hold Back Nothing

Psychoanalysis and Catholicism in Daily Life

I sat in a pew at the back of the sanctuary. Apart from me, there were only a few older women in the pews. The priest had processed into the room with the Eucharist in the monstrance and took his seat as we, together, meditated in the presence of Christ during Holy Hour. I had with me a devotional book with prayers, short essays, and scripture verses to aid me in my meditation. I started to read a poem by St. Francis of Assisi. I read the following line: "Therefore, hold back nothing of yourselves for yourselves, so that He who gives Himself totally to you may receive you totally" (Becklo, 2022, p. 5). I wept. I knew I had been holding back something of myself for myself. In doing so, I had also held back something from God. The consequence was distance from God. This distance was something I had felt for a long time, but I had not realized, until reading this line, that it was my holding back which was responsible for it.

I was responsive to this theological poem because of the work I had done in my personal psychoanalysis. I understood "holding back" in two ways. First, I (my ego) held back from consciousness, i.e. engaged in repression. In fact, holding back parts of myself from myself and from others was a strategy I had employed from a young age to maintain a well-behaved, self-controlled, and pious image of myself.

Second, by "holding back" from consciousness, I inevitably held back from speech. I did not share much of myself, the struggles, concerns, doubts, or sins. Why would I have wanted anyone to know any of those things? When I did speak, the intention was to dispose of those parts, resolve the struggle as soon as possible so I did not have think about them, hold them in consciousness, any longer.

Without these realizations I wrought in psychoanalysis, I would not have been open to the spiritual experience. Without the spiritual experience facilitated by St. Francis and the Eucharist, I would not have been motivated to change. While the issue confronted me during that hour, it was not resolved at the end of the hour. I still had work to do.

This dual need and dual benefit inspired this book. Faith and psychoanalysis do not meet the same need, nor do they perform the same function in my life.

DOI: 10.4324/9781003485346-12

Presumably, when I meet God face to face, I will no longer need psychoanalysis. To a similar extent, the Church as it exists now will no longer be needed in the same form and function. On this side of Heaven, these traditions are central to my ongoing formation as a Catholic and psychologist.

Spiritual and Clinical Origins

I am not a cradle Catholic. However, my first exposure to Catholicism was at a young age. My grandmother was close friends with a deeply Catholic family and would regularly house sit for them. I was invited to sleep over with her. One evening, I was exploring the house. It was mostly a normal house with everything I expected to see.

I eventually opened a door to a room for which I had no model to understand. It was a small, narrow room with a window on the far wall. Along both sides of the room were many statues, icons, crosses, and other devotional materials with a padded kneeler for prayer. I did not understand the purpose of the items but felt in awe of something important. I returned to the room several times over the years when Nana house sat and simply sat and took in the atmosphere.

I grew up in a Protestant environment within the Holiness tradition and had little to no exposure to other Christian denominations or practices. My faith community was framed by services on Sundays and Wednesdays, youth groups and retreats, and camp meetings. It was a low church setting, meaning that there was little formal liturgy and ritual faith practices. The primary activities were small group lessons, contemporary Christian music, and lengthy sermons. I attended mission trips to marginalized communities.

My experience was, not uncommonly, mixed in its impact on me. I deeply benefited from the community and sense of belonging provided by the church. The programs and activities were thoughtful, and the leaders were kind. I generally looked forward to spending time in church. I was instilled with the belief that my relationship with God was personal and I was confident God was invested in my life.

My baptism was the most significant experience of that period. I was in the sixth grade. I went through a several week course at the church to understand what it meant to be baptized. I cannot remember the testimony I provided to the congregation before I was gently immersed in the warm water, but I remember the overwhelming sense of God's love and my connection to all other Christians. There is a picture somewhere in my parent's home of me standing with the pastors. My smile could not have been bigger.

Alongside my positive experience, I also developed a sense that I could not be transparent about my struggles. I internalized an expectation for thoughts and behaviors and did not want to be seen as a sinner. While I witnessed many alter calls, and from time to time went down to the altar myself, I never disclosed the depth of my suffering to anyone.

There was a message that the world outside the church was dangerous to the soul. Each sin was a step closer to hell. Each disclosure of sin was a step outside of the community. I hid as much as I could from others and tried to meet the ideal ego of the young Christian saint, ever frustrated and ashamed that I could not achieve it.

I am not blaming that church, its leaders, or members. While I do hold memories of some damaging messages, my perception and what I internalized of what was taught to me are not to be equated with external reality. It has taken me a long time to understand that dynamic.

My next significant exposure to Catholicism was in college. While I majored in political science, I took an elective course on prayer in the Abrahamic traditions. The course included a retreat to the Abbey of Gethsemane in Kentucky. Thomas Merton, the prolific writer and Trappist monk, resided there from 1941 to his death.

While walking on one of the trails around the monastery, I saw a novice going about his monastic business. He looked to be about my age and his affect was so bright and joyful. I was suddenly struck with confusion and fear. I was in college with a general sense of what I hoped my life would include in the future but no specific sense of myself or who I wanted to be.

Though he had yet to take his vows, here was a man who committed himself to a rule and order for the rest of his life. How did he know, I wondered, that this place was what God wanted for him and what he wanted for himself? I read somewhere that hundreds of men, after reading Merton's (1998) *Seven Story Mountain* when it was first published, ran to join monasteries. I felt a mix of terror, jealousy, and uncertainty.

What did God want for my life? I wanted the clarity I assumed this young novice possessed. Merton's (2011, p. 79) famous prayer became my core spiritual compass.

I planned to attend law school after college. I was enamored with the life and work of Robert F. Kennedy and wanted to become a lawyer like him, educated in the classics but concretely working for the most marginalized people in society. I learned through reading various biographies that he was a devoted Catholic man.

I interned in Washington, D.C. the summer before I graduated college. It was an exhilarating experience. Never had I been so close to what I then considered to be *the action*. I enjoyed the advocacy work, the various lectures by important and powerful people, and experiencing the energy of the crowd outside the Supreme Court when it announced its Obamacare decision.

Yet at the end of the summer, despite all the glamour and excitement, I felt something was missing from the fantasy I had constructed about myself and my future in law and politics. It was no longer a satisfying or motivating image. I entered my senior year of college confused about the future.

I do not have a memory of when it occurred or even in what context. Yet I remember the feeling, the calling from God, to become a pastor. There was no doubt. It was an immense relief and a profound sense of joy. A series of experiences occurred which confirmed the call. I moved across the country and enrolled in a Methodist seminary.

I delved into the study of John Wesley, the founder of Methodism. The most impactful piece of this study came when I read his sermon "The Duty of Constant Communion" (Outler & Heitzenrater, 1991). The title is the clear argument. I learned, contrary to how many of the Wesleyan churches I had attended practiced, that Wesley taught communion should be provided whenever possible.

Wesley played with the language in a way I find relevant to Lacan. "Let every one, therefore, who has either any desire to please God, or any love of his own soul, obey God, and consult the good of his own soul, by *communicating* every time he can" (Outler & Heitzenrater, 1991, p. 504, emphasis added). The Eucharist is the Word, and our engagement with the Word is communication. We are obliged, said Wesley, to communicate as often as we can.

I was not prepared for the shock of the other coursework. So much of what I had been taught to believe as a Christian was challenged during the first few months of the term. Again, I had no prior experience with any other way of thinking. I learned for the first time there were multiple methods of biblical interpretation. I realized this multiplicity of methods did not just apply to scripture; there were many ways of interpreting life, *my* life.

I felt, as I did when I saw the novice, unmoored in my identity and calling. I felt unable to hold a clear, defined image of myself. I felt fraudulent being in the seminary. I needed help. The seminary provided a list of psychotherapists in the area, and I began to see one approximately three months into that first semester.

When I shared with a classmate, someone who had already been pastoring for years, that I started psychotherapy, he asked me, "Isn't Jesus enough?" He was not judgmental; he was entirely sincere.

This question is one of the roots of this book. It is not too far afield from the arguments by Bishop Sheen in the second chapter. All of life, for Sheen and my classmate, was contained and explained in the sin-salvation framework. Whatever irrational struggle I experienced, it was in some way, shape, or form, related to sin. Therefore, the only resource or support which could address that struggle and sin was Jesus and his many clerical workers.

There are many problems with this question. The most important one to me is that everyday experience reveals it to be the wrong question. I wrote in chapter two that Bishop Sheen did not address the reality that many Christians ardently and sincerely participate in the sacraments of the Church and yet struggle within themselves.

They attend mass, they receive the eucharist, they confess their sins and receive absolution, they pray with honesty and earnestness, and they serve the poor and needy. All of that, and many of these Christians experience significant anxiety, depression, mood instability, psychosomatic pain, and many other types of pain.

Isn't Jesus enough? If I said yes, then there would be no point to psychotherapy. If I said no, there would be no point to faith. An immediate question arose in response: enough for what? I began to see a pattern in my life where my ego would consolidate around an Imaginary identity, and I would think to myself: *this is it*.

When I was first introduced to politics and law, I thought *this is it*. This is who I am and what I will do. Everything was clear and known. I sketched out the steps and planned the future. Yet my experience in D.C. confronted me with lack. This was *not* it. That is *not* me. What now?

The image of the novice was important to the recognition of my calling, for my calling provided me with what I assumed, wrongly, the novice possessed. This time, the ego consolidated around divine purpose. *This is it*! Yet my experience in seminary challenged that identity too. This was *not* it. That is *not* me. What now? I briefly considered monastic life. But as one of my professors reminded me, monasteries are not places to hide.

Education and Confirmation

I worked in therapy on this insecurity and shame. I was fortunate to work with a therapist who provided me with space and time to simply talk and share thoughts I had never expressed to anyone without moral judgement or a demand to live a certain way. The reader can probably guess where this story is headed. I concluded, being a therapist, *this is it*! I wanted to be just like my therapist, or at least the image I held of them in my mind.

The pattern repeated. This time, however, I had grown some in my expectations. When I was interviewed for admission to the counseling psychology program, I was clear with the staff that I did not want to commit myself to any clear end. My primary purpose in entering the program was to explore myself, to add theoretical rigor to the personal reflection I was undergoing in therapy.

When I entered seminary, I held clear belief and an idealized image of what I wanted to become. When I entered counseling psychology formation, I had questions. This difference in posture and intent was the inspiration for the seventh chapter of this book. The intent was not to privilege one type of formation over the other but to demonstrate the importance of thinking through the entry, process, and end of formation.

I do not remember what triggered the thought, but near the end of my master's degree, I realized I had no knowledge of Freud other than the basics in any history of psychology course. I was close to graduation and felt I had missed a crucial foundation. There was little primary source reading or teaching about the beginning of psychoanalytic theory and practice.

Few programs that are not explicitly psychoanalytic, and plenty that are, omit Freud from their curriculum. I know this broad omission is a fact. My final semester, I completed an independent project in which I asked the top 100 graduate psychology programs to share whether and how Freud was taught in their programs. With a couple of outliers, it is hard to overstate the mocking responses I received from the faculty.

I started to read Freud from scratch. I wondered if anyone was writing or speaking about Freud today. I googled "Freud today" and learned Bruce Fink (2017) published *A Clinical Introduction to Freud*. Here was a text which provided a comprehensive lesson in Freudian psychoanalysis. Reading the introduction, however, I learned about another psychoanalyst, Jacques Lacan, who returned to Freud and innovated psychoanalytic theory. The first section of this book represents the importance of knowing that foundation.

I read as much as I could of Freud, Lacan, and their many commentators who made sense of and applied their work to contemporary issues. I enlisted a Lacanian supervisor before I graduated to help make sense of my early clinical work with case management and have continued meeting with them since then. I was hungry for more understanding and training. I pursued a doctorate in clinical psychology at school which was primarily psychoanalytic in its orientation.

Meanwhile, having left seminary, I searched for a new church. My internal disillusionment projected onto my church experiences. I felt self-righteousness and arrogant about my criticisms of the churches I attended. I did not know where to go. Eugene Peterson recommended, in a book I cannot remember, to look for the smallest, closest church and commit oneself there for a year.

As it happened, the closest church to me, though not small, was a Catholic parish. I sat at the back of the church and listened to the sermon, knelt and stood, knelt and stood, and received a blessing during the liturgy of the Eucharist. There was no profound single moment, but I felt the liturgy drew me to humble myself in ways that did not induce shame. I was not in the center. The priest was not in the center. The Eucharist was in the center.

I eventually contacted the parish office and requested information on confirmation. I began the Rite of Christian Initiation for Adults (RCIA). The meetings I attended each week with fellow candidates and catechumens were rich in conversation and learning. Our facilitator was a woman around my age who was sharp, smart, and passionate. I was engaged at all levels of my being, intellectual, spiritual, psychological, and more.

During Holy Thursday of Easter week, those of us in the RCIA process were invited to have our feet washed by our priest, as Jesus did for his disciples during the Last Supper. It is hard to describe in words what that experience was like for me. I cried. There is no correlate in the psychoanalytic process. The picture taken of me that night shows my face as dumbfounded. This act of service and humility goes far beyond the desire of the analyst and touches the Real.

During Good Friday, as a group, we carried the cross. Freud, as I quoted in the first chapter, considered transference to be a cross. Though he may have just been poetic about a general sense of burden, I think we can understand his reflection as a recognition of the humility required of the analyst. The joke with clergy who wear the white collar is that the little white tab is a small screen onto which people can project whatever they want. For the period of the session, the person of the analyst is not centered, not known.

Freud and Lacan often relied on religious terminology to help make sense of their clinical experiences and theories. They recognized their work was about more than cure, more than about health or illness, more than about behavior and its antecedents and consequences. That "more" is hard to describe using positivist, scientific language. Religious signifiers offer a depth of meaning necessary to understanding psychoanalytic experience, as analyst and analysand.

My experience of the Easter Vigil was similar to my baptism. When I received the Eucharist for the first time as a Catholic, I felt more joy than I can describe. My confirmation name is St. (and Doctor of the Church) Irenaeus. Because of his writing to clarify theology against early heresies, Irenaeus is considered the patron saint of theologians and catechists. I would simplify the list and say he is the patron saint of truth. I pray for his intercession that I may encounter truth, about myself, about the Other, about God.

When it came time for internship, I moved across the country (again). For the first time in nearly eight years, I was not in psychotherapy. I lived near a monastery and learned the monks there offered spiritual direction. I began spiritual direction once a month while I completed my fulltime training at an inpatient state psychiatric hospital. This site was not my first choice. I interviewed with several other sites closer to home and was turned down by each one. Again, I was confused and uncertain.

I gradually learned during these spiritual direction meetings that the way I previously considered discernment and vocation were self-centered. Such a conception ignored the context in which God places us. I missed, until then, the role of the Other. My discernment attempted clarity and knowledge and therefore ignored the unconscious, that which I could not know. First, I needed to accept that I decided to be there. I needed to accept where I was, in terms of geography and clinical placement. I needed to decide that where I was, who I was with, and what I was doing was meaningful.

This meaning was derived from my spiritual beliefs. I could say, though I could not know, that God would shape me and those around me with this new experience. However, the attribution of meaning need not be divine purpose. To assume meaning in what could otherwise be considered insignificant is a psychoanalytic act. Analysts do not know what a dream means in any objective sense, but they assume there is latent and manifest content to explore. They encourage the patient to explore this meaning. My spiritual director pushed me to explore the significance of my decisions, my placement, and my work. That year was one of the most fruitful experiences of my life.

Intersections of Catholicism and Psychoanalysis

I returned home and decided it was time to enter Lacanian psychoanalysis proper. I told the analyst that I wanted the experience to better understand theory, improve my clinical work, and, with some hesitation, I said I needed to address relationship problems. The analyst told me that it was good I had identified the third goal, as the first two would not have been sufficient reasons to begin analysis. Psychoanalysis is not a purely intellectual pursuit. As I wrote in chapter seven, analysis requires a symptom. What is not working?

St. Francis said to hold back nothing. This command is not far from Freud's fundamental rule of free association. I wrote the second section of the book based on theological and theoretical concepts which circulated around this evident demand for holding nothing back and my longstanding pattern of holding what I perceived to be bad thoughts and desires within myself. I grew up in a church setting which seemed to communicate the opposite of what St. Francis asked of Christians. The Catholic Church, historically, practiced extensive censorship, as illustrated in the first and fourth chapters.

While I do not agree with everything Maryse Choisy, Angelo Hesnard, and Marc Oraison wrote, I strongly believe their voices should have been encouraged, not censored. Those who question the church, like the hysteric's discourse in chapter eight, provide an opportunity to develop and reveal further knowledge. Holding back that discourse only hurts the Church and others who might benefit from hearing it.

What I found compelling about the work of Choisy was her lifelong attention to people on the margins. She wanted to give these people an opportunity and a medium through which to be heard. I believe Pope Francis would have appreciated this posture as well. Yet the Church chose to censor her because her ideas and opinions did not perfectly align with the Magisterium at the time. The Holy Office thought her work was dangerous yet did not see the danger when they censored her necessary questions.

Angelo Hesnard was a complicated figure in French psychoanalysis. Yet his emphasis on the practical, tangible consequences of behavior remains important when thinking through ethics and moral law. When the Church maintains a moral law that only carries a seemingly spiritual consequence, then people do not have a reason beyond avoiding internal guilt to obey to it. Caught in a complicated web of spiritual moral laws and internal conflict about whether to adhere to them, people are no longer attentive to reality outside of their minds. Such a system does not lead people to holiness or to contributing to the Kingdom of God.

Marc Oraison, as I wrote in chapter four, seemed to distinguish between sin and symptom. He did not use this language; it is my interpretation of his work. I do not think this distinction has received the attention it deserves since Beirnaert (1951) wrote "Does Sanctification Depend on Psychic Structure?" Beirnaert rightly concluded, no. But we need further discussion to deepen our understanding of this tension between sin and symptom. Oraison seemed to make the definition of mortal sin so specific as to almost be non-existent. The critical reviewers of his text took him to mean that without sin, people are not responsible for their actions, that psychic conflict absolves an individual of responsibility. I do not think this is what Oraison meant, but the full explanation has yet to be explored in detail.

Chapter five, on Rahner and Lacan, was my attempt at a beginning to this exploration. Freedom is restricted by sin and symptom. Freedom is the goal of spiritual and psychoanalytic development. Unlike Hesnard, I think we still need the term and notion of sin. Why? Because it helps us understand the responsibility we hold for our symptoms. Psychoanalysis is almost alone in the models of psychopathology and treatment in this regard. Symptoms are a complex interplay of fate and responsibility and are inherently moral issues. We are not responsible for our history, our Symbolic coordinates, but we are responsible for how we respond to them.

I needed a way to accept my responsibility for my desires and decisions that did not exacerbate the harsh judgment of my superego. Holding only to a notion of sin, especially in a purely judicial-behavioral framework, only exacerbates that judgment. In the Church, that is the source of the infamous Catholic guilt and the scrupulosity which can result from it. One need only look online today and see the unfortunate number of Catholic people who post questions along the lines of "Is [insert desire or behavior] a sin?" or "Was it a sin for my priest to [insert opinion or behavior]?" The questions on sin and sexuality are especially prevalent.

The framework of "sin or not" is a strictly legal question. It is not, fundamentally, a spiritual question. Presumably, if the person receives a sentence of sin, they feel guilt, go to confession and seek absolution, and perform penance. If they receive a sentence of not sin, they do not need to feel guilty and do not need to perform any confession or penance. This determination does not address the unconscious, the desire underneath the desire or action. Such a legal conclusion closes a conversation rather than opening up further reflection. This adjudication was part of the obsessive rituals Freud identified in Catholicism.

I remember one of the first times I went to confession with my priest. I began to list the various sins I thought I needed to confess. My priest asked me, "Adam, why are you here?" I was a little confused. I thought my presence was self-evident. This encounter is the sacrament of reconciliation, I thought, I am not here to get my tires changed. But what the priest asked of me was for me to articulate for myself what was not working in my life. Listing offenses to canon law does not communicate that level of confession.

The question, "Why are you here?" informed my participation in psychoanalysis. It also informed my clinical practice. It is a central question for the process of psychoanalysis overall and for each session. The need for psychoanalysis, for reconciliation, for spiritual direction, for faith, is not self-evident. Both contexts are rooted in original sin as articulated by Rahner and original desire as articulated by Lacan.

I started this reflection with my experience in adoration. Following this tumultuous experience, I visited with my priest to discuss my experience and wrestle with what to do with the parts of myself that I held back from everyone. He advised me to write a letter to allow me the time and space to craft what I needed to say. I was struck, but not surprised, that I received no moral judgment. I was encouraged to speak. Doing so radically changed my life. While I am not done with psychoanalysis or faith, I am freer with my decisions.

Faith, reason, and the unconscious. I ended the third chapter with the argument that these terms represent the *three* orders of knowledge that must be recognized today. This argument is theoretical, clinical, and phenomenological. The Church still needs to take account of the unconscious. Psychoanalysis needs to better understand the necessity of faith to the psyche (not restricted to Catholicism). These three orders of knowledge are required to develop and use interior freedom. As Jacques Phillipe (2002, p. 37) wrote, "When we see ourselves with God's eyes, we experience tremendous freedom. It could be called a double freedom: to be sinners, and to become saints."

This dual freedom is represented as far back as the story of Oedipus. The gay Catholic poet John Martin Finlay (2020) wrote "Two Poems for Oedipus." The first read:

> You blind King Oedipus, emblem of mind,
> In whom Apollo sunk those awful claws,
> No fate forced you to learn your crimes.
> The god left free kinetic intellect,
> Deathless, matterless, itself like god,
> Which cuts like acid to a final cause.
> You chose and seized yourself the agony
> Of kingship, goat-song of purest law.
> Unshadowed noon, the isolated throne,
> Clearing of marble lit by reason's god –
> You held these blinded in your sacrifice.
> (Finlay, 2020, p. 52)

I earlier described the tension between fate and responsibility. Finlay tells us no fate forced Oedipus to learn his crimes. He chose and seized himself the agony of kingship. He was free to be a sinner and a saint. His kinetic intellect (reason), his faith (sacrifice), and unconscious (blinded) together moved Oedipus forward past fate into responsible freedom.

Ending

While I was writing this book, Pope Francis died. This loss was difficult for me. For the duration of my Catholic faith until then, I knew no other Holy Father. His generosity of spirit welcomed me into the Church. It was his pastoral heart and practice which helped me see the connections between Catholic faith and psychoanalytic theory and practice. From his emphasis on accompaniment, to the apostolate of the ear, his desire to move the Church closer to the margins, showing mercy not sacrifice, synodality, and so much more, Pope Francis instituted a new discourse in the papacy and the Church. Not new, exactly, but a return to the pastoral dimensions of the early church. I admit, I was not ready for this ending when it came.

Pope Francis should be remembered for how he taught us to remember, experience, and share God's love for all of creation, from people to the planet and every detail in between. He gave his last public breaths pointing us, again, to the resurrection of Jesus and the power of love over death. In a world that is so divided by hate, I pray for the strength, determination, and heart to carry on this work of love in my life.

Freud once referred to education and psychoanalysis as impossible professions. To that add we should add the papacy and indeed all of clerical life. While I critically analyzed the speech of Pope Francis in the eighth chapter using Lacan's four discourses, Pope Francis did the best he could to address billions of people in different roles, positions, places, and with varied histories. His papacy, as his name, stands alone.

My partner and I had the opportunity to see Pope Francis during a general audience when I was in Rome in September 2024 conducting research for this book. He had just returned from his apostolic journey to Indonesia, Papua New Guinea, Timor-Leste, and Singapore. He shared with the crowd in Rome, "A first reflection that comes naturally after this journey is that in thinking of the Church, we are still too Eurocentric, or as they say, 'western.' But in reality, *the Church is much bigger*, much bigger than Rome and Europe, much bigger!" (Francis, 2024, para. 3).

This reflection is also the most significant limitation of this book. With brief references as exceptions, I have written a Western book on Catholicism and psychoanalysis. If one wants to find a strong intersection between Catholicism and psychoanalysis, Latin America is the obvious location. The deep well of liberation theology promises important implications for psychoanalytic theory and I hope to familiarize myself with this literature and seeing more in the future (see, for example, Gaztambide, 2015). The Eastern Church is another region and tradition which is worth exploring at length (as Waitz & Tisdale, 2022, and Cazacu, 2013, have done well).

Pope Leo XIV now leads the Catholic Church. I fervently pray that with his leadership, the Church once again seeks dialogue with psychoanalysis. There are too many issues today which require the three orders of knowledge to address. I am confident Freud's secular pastoral worker (the psychoanalyst) and the Catholic religious (men and women) can work together not to judge or diagnosis, but to accompany and encourage the speech of the many suffering people in our world today.

References

Becklo, M. (2022). *The holy hour: Meditations for eucharistic adoration.* Word on Fire.

Beirnaert, L. (1951). Does sanctification depend on psychic structure? *CrossCurrents,* 1 (2): 39–43. (J. Caulfield, Trans.). (Original work published 1950)

Cazacu, P. (2013). *Orthodoxy and psychoanalysis: Dirge or polychronion to the centuries-old tradition?* Peter Lang GbmH.

Fink, B. (2017). *A clinical introduction to Freud: Techniques for everyday practice.* Norton.

Finlay, J.M. (2020). *"Dense poems & socratic light": The poetry of John Martin Finlay (1941–1991).* D. Middleton & J.P. Doucet (Eds.). Wiseblood Books.

Francis. (2024). General audience: Wednesday, September 18, 2024. Vatican. https://www.vatican.va/content/francesco/en/audiences/2024/documents/20240918-udienza-generale.html.

Gaztambide, D. (2015). A preferential option for the repressed: Psychoanalysis through the eyes of liberation theology. *Psychoanalytic Dialogues,* 25(6). doi:10.1080/10481885.2015.1097281.

Merton, T. (1998). *The seven story mountain: An autobiography of faith.* Harcourt, Inc.

Merton, T. (2011). *Thoughts in solitude.* Farrar, Straus and Giroux.

Outler, A. & Heitzenrater, R. (1991). *John Wesley's sermons: An anthology.* Abingdon Press.

Phillipe, J. (2002). *Interior freedom.* (H. Scott, Trans.). Scepter Publishers, Inc.

Waitz, C. & Tisdale, T. (2022). *Lacanian psychoanalysis and eastern orthodox Christian anthropology in dialogue.* Routledge.

Index

For Product Safety Concerns and Information please contact our
EU representative GPSR@taylorandfrancis.com Taylor & Francis
Verlag GmbH, Kaufingerstraße 24, 80331 München, Germany